# Getting REAL About Alzheimer's

## **R**ementia Through **E**ngagement, **A**ssistance, and **L**ove

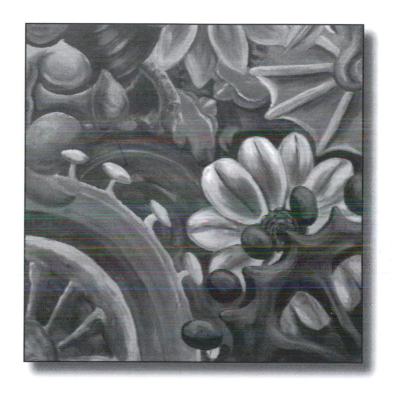

Kassandra A. King, BA, NHA, RCFE

**Plain View Press, LLC**
http://plainviewpress.net

1011 W 34th Street, STE 404
Austin, TX 78705

ISBN: 978-1-63210-004-7
Library of Congress Control Number: 2014942676


Cover art *Wagon Wheels and Flowers* by Thor Harris with permission
Cover design by Pam Knight

## Acknowledgements

A world of gratitude and love for your support, editing, interest, encouragement, and patience: to Pam Knight, Publisher, Plainview Press, thank you for sharing the vision, taking a chance on me, and the gentle nudges to finish my manuscript; to my readers and editors: Roger Krueger, Russel Ray, Peter Nilsson, Melissa Stinson, Magdalena Lederer, and Mary Jo Robb for your time, compliments and criticisms; to Paul Marangella and Josh Buller for the opportunity that gave me the inspiration to write this book; Dr. Tom Kitwood (deceased) for his brilliant writings on rementia theory; Julian Rey Saenz and Wende Chan for proofing and to Dorothy Knight for reading, editing, and for instilling in me, by her own example, compassion for those with unmet needs.

Author can be reached through Alzheimer's Connection La Mesa, www.alzconnectlamesa.com

# Contents

## Section 1: Rementia

## Section 2: Engagement

# Section 3: Assistance

# Section 4: Love

# References

*to caregivers everywhere*
*and to those whom they love*

# Getting REAL About Alzheimer's

Rementia through Engagement, Assistance, and Love

## Introduction

Recently I was hosting a guest from a country where extended families commonly live together: grandparents, cousins, aunts, and uncles, along with his own parents, brothers, and sisters. His family shared an apartment complex occupied by only his relatives—36 family members in one location. When I explained my career in long-term care and my special attention to those with Alzheimer's disease (AD), he told me his Grandfather has Alzheimer's. He said he did not think it should be called a disease because most old people have it. Why is it a problem? I pointed out the difference between family living arrangements in his country and ours, and then he understood.

In the United States and in other countries, most families are fragmented and spread across cities, states, and in other countries. *Professional caregivers come to the rescue.* We fill in when family or friends are unavailable or unable. Persons with forms of dementia have huge needs—day after day, night after night. Only a small percentage of the work force chooses to attempt the direct caregiver job, which has expectations beyond what a mortal should be asked to do. The public and the media have been unkind to us, airing stories about abusive caregivers and poor conditions. Rarely does anyone bring up the positive impact we make in lives.

We have come so far from what I saw during my first nursing home visit 35 years ago. I recall the dank, odorous hallways where residents were lined up, slumped over in their wheelchairs. Regulations and training requirements have served this population well. Protocols have been implemented with good results. Today, the majority of care communities are clean, well-lit places to live or receive rehabilitation.

My volunteer career began in middle school with my family participating in a nationwide effort—"The Holiday Project." Hundreds of people gathered on Christmas day and made visits to hospitals and nursing homes, singing carols and distributing small gifts. In high school choir, we gave Christmas performances in nursing homes. While most students made a beeline for the door after the performance, I lingered behind, talking to the residents. The bodily fluids, food-smeared faces and distressed moans did not deter me.

I wanted to connect.

After college, I joined a volunteer group doing weekly visits to a nursing home. After the group broke up, I continued to go. One day I was in the dining room visiting Goldie, whom I had grown quite fond of and taken out for ice cream and to the plant nursery. As was often the case, the trays were brought out in the big silver rolling cart with no staff in sight. I knew many of the residents by name, so I took it upon myself to begin passing the food trays.

A nicely dressed man entered the room and asked who I was. He advised me that I needed special training and approval from the director of nursing to pass trays. He was an administrator in training at the nursing home. Somehow by the end of the conversation, he had convinced me to enter a post-graduate program to become a licensed nursing home administrator. Two years later, I sat at the desk of my first nursing home, head in my hands thinking, "What am I supposed to do about this?" Like parenthood, no amount of study, apprenticeship, advice, or volunteering prepares a person for the immense and intense role of nursing home administrator. The worst aspect of the job was the lack of time for interaction with residents. Not the right match for me.

Early in my career, I became fascinated with Alzheimer's disease (AD). People with AD are enjoyable to be with, albeit at times tough to please. They are refreshing to me because most are no longer attempting to impress anyone. They are genuine. Relating to the true essence of someone with dementia feels natural to me.

This book was largely inspired by my recent experience as program manager of engagement (activities) in a very large assisted living memory care community. Day after day, I worked on creating new and meaningful programs based on person-centered care philosophy. The company president had great respect for the book "Dementia Reconsidered" by Dr. Thomas Kitwood. He challenged me to read the book and "transform" the way activities were being conducted. In the book, the term "rementia" describes bringing individuals back into meaningful forms of participation in daily life. Rementia is a term more commonly heard in the United Kingdom than in the United States, but it is becoming meaningful here, too.

For six months, I developed programs and trained the staff on engagement and person-centered care philosophy. What I experienced was profound, exciting and, at times, breathtaking (especially when I followed a caregiver's suggestion to have residents play badminton!) By emphasizing resident choice and variety in programming, residents who formerly stated throughout the day, "I want to go home," instead asked what we were going to do next. Through implementing a modular system and encouraging personhood, the community was transformed into a place where residents were in charge of how their time was spent. Staff members were encouraged to express individual talents and to play, entertain, and bring a sense of freedom to the environment.

Care communities have changed immensely since I entered the field professionally two decades ago. In 1998, I wrote a published article entitled "Abracadabra, Can You Be Restraint Free?" (Long-Term Care News, Spring 1998). At the time, restraint reduction was regarded as extremely difficult—maybe even impossible. We thought it would be too dangerous conforming to new regulations, set at zero tolerance. Now, the thought of using a vest restraint to prevent someone from falling out of a wheelchair seems absurd. In this book, I am proposing we loosen the psychological restraints society has placed on persons with dementia. Maybe someday not allowing residents to assist preparing their meals will seem absurd. Presently, that idea is quite a stretch. However, we can make major changes in engagement programming and how we view persons with memory loss.

We used to call areas for people at risk of leaving the premises "lock down units." Imagine the horror of a resident with mild dementia overhearing that he is staying in the lock down unit. Now we most commonly call these "secure units." Can we master the techniques of person-centered care and drastically reduce the risk of resident elopement by doing so? If residents have a sense of purpose in the care community, the urge to leave may be eliminated.

## Getting REAL

This book is about practical possibilities. In *Getting REAL About Alzheimer's* I am *proposing a shift* in beliefs that contribute to the downward spiral of dementia. I know a shift is possible because I have seen it happen. And the difference is huge. I know this from personal experience, observations and knowledge. I am a volunteer turned administrator, educator and care consultant. I am not a doctor, licensed nurse or therapist. I write from direct involvement with thousands of caregivers and care receivers, and from ideas of other experts that confirm my vision of possibility with rementia. From lessons learned, these pages contain practical solutions to widespread problems.

This book is a guide for family and friends of people with Alzheimer's, as well as for professional caregivers. It is my gift to the residents in care communities who have always seen the best in me, and who continue to give me unconditional love. It is my hope that this book will help others who are giving and receiving love through the services they provide. When I reference "*REAL*" or "*Getting REAL*" in this book, I am referring to the philosphy of Rementia through Engagement, Assistance, and Love. May we get closer to *REAL* each and every day.

**R**ementia through

**E**ngagement,

**A**ssistance, and

**L**ove

## TILT Keys

Following each section is a set of questions about the content. These topics are part of my *Training Insights for Learning Transformation* (TILT) program. The questions help individuals examine issues and observe their own thinking in a new light. In a classroom setting these questions generate group discussion and reveal caregiver viewpoints.

Although this guide is written in a format that highlights caregivers in community settings, it is fully intended to be just as helpful to family members and friends. Those who want to know more about how to care for their loved ones can equally learn how to provide meaningful options for those with impaired mental states.

It is most effective for those using this guide to complete the TILT sections once as they study the material, and then again after reading the entire book. Comparing answers will be a good measure of increased understanding.

# Section 1: Rementia

## What Is Rementia?

Mr. Williams approached me, holding a worn piece of notebook paper. His hands trembled slightly as he gripped the edges of the paper. Written in blue highlighter was a list of names and phone numbers, those of his adult children. He asked if it was time to call his son. I had just started working at the assisted living where he had been residing for about two months. Upon reviewing the list, I noticed someone had written next to the son's name "gets home from teaching school at 4:30." The time was now 2:00.

Though I am not a doctor, nurse, or licensed clinician, I am familiar with the signs of anxiety, and Mr. Williams appeared quite anxious and uncomfortable. He wore a heavy winter coat with a sweater and shirt underneath although he stayed indoors. The weather was perfect—October, Southern California. I advised him it would be another 2 ½ hours before his son would be home. For the next 2 ½ hours I saw Mr. Williams pacing in the area outside of my office, holding the notebook paper, asking staff what time it was and if it was time to call his son yet. He would go into his room for a few minutes and come back out. Mr. Williams has the diagnosis of Alzheimer's disease, thus he has short term memory loss. Therefore, he would not remember he had asked before asking again nor could he remember what time it was from minute to minute.

During the waiting period, I asked if he would like to go outside. He said it was too cold. A pianist was performing in the dining room. He was not inclined to join the audience. His sole focus was calling his son. This call was the highlight of every day.

For many days, I observed the pattern. Mr. Williams would dwell in the area near the phone, holding his list—the lifeline to his identity. Every day he wore the thick coat with multiple layers of clothing, saying he was cold. My attempts to get him involved in group activities were futile.

One day I convinced him to step outside into the garden patio with me. At first he said he was cold and would like to go back inside. I knew from talking to his son that Mr. Williams used to enjoy gardening, so I showed him the flowers I had brought to start a gardening project. The grounds had not received much attention from the professional gardeners, and the executive director had given me permission to do whatever possible with the area. I asked Mr. Williams to help me plant the flowers, telling him my boss wanted me to start the project.

Mr. Williams asked where I would like to plant the flowers. I asked him for suggestions. Thus began the rementia process for Mr. Williams. In the beginning, Mr. Williams would ask where to plant the flowers, though I always asked his opinion and went along with his ideas. One day he asked if we could pull out the miscellaneous vines and growth to make room for more flowers. "Absolutely!" I responded. So, he began doing weeding and uprooting, clearing large areas.

After a few weeks of work, off came the coat!

When we bagan the project I would need to remind Mr. Williams to water the plants every day, asking politely if he could be responsible for making sure we kept the ground moist. He would ask each day "Where is the hose?" and I would point out the spout behind a bush. Soon he began watering every day without reminders. Each day when I arrived on the job, he would be waiting for me to ask what else he should do in the garden.

Then I realized Mr. Williams was no longer carrying the phone list nor was he asking when he could call his son. Instead, he was asking me when I was going to the nursery for more plants. I could hardly keep up with his desire to garden—one day I purchased five six packs of annuals, and he had them in the ground before the day was over! He did not even ask where to plant them. His independent judgment skills had returned! On another day, he spread four large bags of fertilized soil evenly throughout the garden. A conscientious and hard working man, he always washed the spades and shovels after use, putting them back where they belonged. And he always rolled up the hose after watering. His quality of work was equal to, if not better than, any hired professional.

Within a few months, everyone was noticing the lovely results of Mr. Williams' efforts. Daily he requested I come out to the garden to see how the flowers were doing and to ask what I thought about expanding into another area we had yet to touch. He also asked if "the big guys" were happy with his work. Of course they were! And they told him so as well.

In the garden there were four old holly berry bushes—the type impossible to kill—taking up precious planting space, and Mr. Williams was ready to take them out. This was no easy task, and I was concerned he might be overdoing it. So, I checked with others in decision making positions, and we all agreed to let him try.

And then, off came the sweater!

Amazing! Mr. Williams was dedicated to getting the project done, but I chose to limit his digging to one bush per day. During the removal of the shrubs, I did stand by to ensure he maintained his balance and was not putting himself at risk. He never fell. He had zero injuries. He knew what he was doing and how to do it. When spring came, I was bringing sprouts of asylum and forget-me-nots (a nice coincidence) from my own yard weekly. Mr. Williams and several other residents helped me to carry pots from my Jeep.

By April, the patio garden was eye catching. Mr. Williams and another strong resident put in stepping stones. Several residents had been participating in planting and pulling out weeds and vines, and one day Mr. Williams said to me, "See how when we get all these people we get so much done working together?" Many times I got teary eyed sharing the joy of what was accomplished in the garden.

Mr. Williams found a new life of purpose, where he spent his days doing meaningful work. *Rementia—a return to the wellness of the mind.* He had a project that meant a lot to him, to me, and to everyone who spent time in the patio garden. Though he received compliments left and right, he was a humble man who would divert the recognition from himself by making jokes.

Even in the middle of the winter—though in Southern California—I would find him out in the garden in a T-shirt.

"Mr. Williams—please come in and put on your coat!" I would say.

"I don't need my coat. I feel just fine," he would reply.

To be "remented" is to experience re-establishment of the individual self: to hold beliefs, practice values and have freedom of expression. Just as a person who has had an accident resulting in physical injury can be rehabilitated through physical therapy and support from others, a person who has experienced a decline due to dementia can be remented to a new level of active and joyful living.

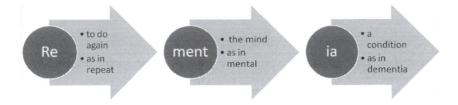

**Figure 1.1** Rementia In Syllables

**re**—to do again, such as in the words, repeat, return, relive, reverse, retrieve, and re-set
**ment**—having to do with the mind
**ia**— a state of being or condition

A person who is remented has been returned to an awareness of who he is and his capabilities. Whether or not the person has returned to the same state of mind prior to dementia is not the purpose of rementia. The goal is transformation of a person from a state of helpless, hopeless and useless to a person who is capable, willing and helpful.

Throughout this book I will be referencing the writings of Dr. Tom Kitwood in the incredible book *Dementia Reconsidered*. Dr. Kitwood is credited for defining the keys to rementia—*person-centered care* and *personhood*. Before reading Dr. Kitwood's book, I had not heard the term rementia, but I had seen it happen in residents even prior to Mr. Williams and the garden. The book reaffirmed my belief in the possibility of bringing out the best in each and every resident. Dr. Kitwood's philosophy matches my own with regard to the social aspects of living and each person's "unique way of experiencing life and relationships." (Dr. Kitwood, viii)

## Personhood and Person-Centered Care

Just as each person has a unique self before they have signs of dementia, a person remains unique during all stages of dementia. Personality is an individual trait. Four residents who share a table in the dining room may have the same clinical diagnosis and may have similar limitations in caring for themselves. That does not mean they share the same needs, wants and desires. As caregivers, we must avoid the tendency to group people together and assume they will all like the same entertainment, daily schedule, room temperature, or foods.

If we go about caregiving without considering what is special about each person we care for, we do not support each as whole human beings. Though it sounds awful, residents are often seen as objects to which a service must be performed. Even the best caregivers fall into the habit of 'doing' without seeing a person with a rich history, preferences, individual thoughts and feelings. In the course of a busy day full of tasks, caregivers can easily fall into the trap of thinking solely about getting the job done. True caregiving includes a focus on *how the job is being done*.

Culture change is a term used in skilled nursing care that refers to providing services according to individual likes and dislikes. Person-centered care and culture change contain very similar ideas. Readers who have been exposed to culture change practices have a good foundation for continuing to learn about person-centered care. There are several terms for person-centered care: patient centered, resident centered, person directed, and relationship centered.

Honoring personhood goes deeper than acknowledging whether or not someone prefers a shower in the morning or evening. Although respecting preferences in personal grooming is certainly very important, having "authentic contact and communication" (Dr. Kitwood 4) should be first on the to-do list during each busy shift. Section 3 of this guide explores methods of person-centered care while assisting with activities of daily living.

At the core of rementia, the connection made between those who are caregivers and those receiving the care is personal. Do you know the essence of *who she is?* Can you see her personality, her beauty, her spirit? Are you showing yours?

A person with dementia is suffering from a change in mental ability: primarily, the memory does not retain or recall information well enough to live as he did prior to the onset of dementia symptoms. The memory loss is accompanied by difficulty making decisions, completing tasks, and handling daily responsibilities. Due to a loss of functionality, many persons with dementia are experiencing a drastic reduction in social relationships accompanied by a loss of identity.

"I just don't feel like myself," and "I used to know what to do," are words often heard from a person with dementia. A woman who makes such statements has lost footing on the ground of her own personhood. Her sense of self becomes less firm as time passes. Dementia is mental quicksand. A caregiver is a member of the rescue team that prevents her from sinking. If we fail to pull her out from the darkness of dementia, she disappears altogether. We use person-centered care to get her back on solid ground.

15

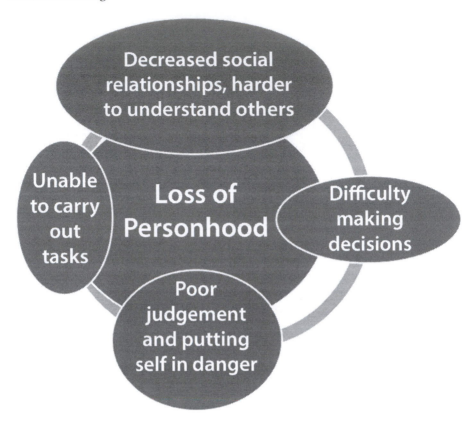

**Figure 1.2** Loss of Personhood

## About Dementia

What is dementia? Though readers of this book may be acquainted with many diseases and conditions that cause dementia symptoms, a brief review of the three most common, from my experience in long-term care settings, is presented herein. Dementia is a broad term used to describe a condition of limited mental capabilities. Some forms of dementia are progressive, some are not. A person who has one type may be able to carry out the same tasks from diagnosis until time of death. In some cases skills may gradually decrease, while in others deterioration happens quickly. Understanding the varieties of dementia is helpful to grasp how the concept of rementia applies in each individual case.

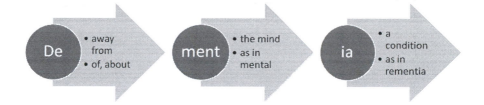

**Figure 1.3** Dementia In Syllables

**de**—Away from or about, such as in the words depart, deduct, detail, defeat and deceive
**ment**—of the mind
**ia**—a state of being or condition

Thus, dementia describes a person who is "out of his mind." The word demented is not a nice way to describe a person struggling with cognitive impairment. Dementia is not a medical diagnosis, although people commonly believe so. The term dementia is used to describe characteristics such as:

- memory loss
- inability to carry out tasks
- poor judgment and decision making

There are many types of dementia; however, the three most prevalent forms I have worked with in long-term care are Alzheimer's disease, cerebral vascular dementia (following a stroke or other brain injury), and Parkinsonian/Lewy Body type dementia. A combination of these conditions can occur, making it even harder to gauge a person's abilities.

Again for the record, I am not a licensed clinician. I am a licensed nursing home administrator with a comprehensive work history that includes dementia care education and training. I am writing from my personal experience and knowledge in order to propose helpful methods of working with individuals who have forms of dementia.

## Alzheimer's Disease

Alzheimer's disease (AD) accounts for approximately half of the cases of dementia. It is estimated that 50 percent of persons over the age of 85 exhibit the signs and symptoms of AD (www.sanalz.org). There are two types of AD: one occurs in persons age 65 and older, and the other, known as Early Onset, can strike as early as the late twenties. Alzheimer's disease is characterized by a profound loss of memory and is usually a very long and progressive illness. AD is a terminal illness and there is no cure or known way to stop the course of the disease. On the average, 8-11 years from the time of diagnosis the decrease in brain function results in major organ failure and death.

Alzheimer's disease symptoms are often grouped into three stages, and sometimes those stages are broken into several different levels. With regard to engagement and ability, there is a wide range of comprehension in persons considered "early stage" and "middle stage." Therefore, the stages are generalizations that could be a contributing factor in *not fully meeting the engagement needs* of persons with AD. If we read in a chart that a person is classified as middle stage we may assume he is not going to be able to follow a step by step process. Likewise, we may believe a person in early stage is capable of higher skill level activities than he is currently demonstrating. Further complicating the assessment process is the tendency for people with AD to have good days and lesser days, with significant changes in clarity and focus.

For the purpose of describing the phases, I will follow the standard language of early (beginning, mild), middle (intermediate, moderate), and late (advanced, severe). The staging method is useful to explain what is expected to happen. And, persons may display signs from one or all of the stages simultaneously.

Characteristics of Early Stage:

- Memory loss becomes apparent
- Takes longer to complete tasks
- Working memory affected—forgetting steps in process
- Difficulty managing money, decreased reasoning ability
- Mood changes
- Increased anxiety, fixated on certain wants/needs/ideas
- Confusion in familiar places
- Operating electronic devices, such as telephones, remote controls, appliances, and computers, may become challenging

Persons in the early stage are often in good physical health. The majority whom I have cared for had no other diagnosis and took very little, if any, medications other than those prescribed to lessen the symptoms of AD. A person with early AD may seem like any other person during short conversations. Social skills and manners usually stay intact throughout the early stages.

Characteristics of Middle Stage:

- Language is affected—word searching, incomplete sentences
- Social skills such as manners and courtesy may disappear—may become inappropriate
- Physical ability starts to decline—difficulty with larger body movements
- Unsure of weekday, month, year, previous homesteads, time periods
- Unaware of conscious thoughts, losing track of flow in conversations
- May begin "wandering" ( what I call "searching")
- Shows agitation more easily
- May be suspicious or paranoid or even have hallucinations
- Repetitive statements and/or movements (such as nodding head over and over)
- May have incontinent episodes
- May begin confusing strangers for familiar people and vice versa
- Instinctive behavior is strong—need for safety, nourishment, sexual tendencies

The middle stage is usually the longest phase. Persons may stay at a particular level of functioning for extended periods of time without major changes. Skill level with self-care varies, as will ability to participate in activities that require focusing or creativity. Concentration for long periods (such as watching a movie) becomes difficult. The "filter" with regard to what is acceptable in public becomes thin. During this stage, a person may be "time traveling," speaking from a place of memory and seeking familiar persons and places and belongings that have been absent from daily life for many years.

Characteristics of Late Stage:

- Does not seem to recognize family, loved ones, close friends
- Verbal communication is minimal—unable to effectively express needs or converse
- May yell, scream, moan loudly
- Unable to care for self on many levels
- Appears disconnected from environment
- Has lost large motor skills control—unable to walk or reposition self
- No control of bowel and bladder
- Instinctive behavior disappears (stops eating)

Persons in late stage become 'bed bound' or 'wheelchair bound.' Appetite is absent and nourishment is obtained only with assistance from others. Providing assistance with bathing, grooming and incontinent care can be very challenging and often persons in this stage may be combative when receiving assistance. Hospice services can be very helpful at this time.

## Vascular Dementia

One cause of vascular dementia is a cerebral vascular accident (CVA), commonly known as a stroke, and is due to blood clotting in vessels of the brain. Aneurysms (bulging) and other problems in circulation that affect oxygen flow can also cause vascular dementia. Physical impairment varies greatly depending on the severity and location of brain tissue damage. There may be paralysis, loss of bowel and bladder control, and other outward physical problems.

Symptoms of vascular dementia include but are not limited to short term memory loss, word searching, confusion, frequent tearfulness or excessive laughter, verbal outbursts, inappropriate social conduct, and rapid mood changes. Several residents I have known with vascular dementia were prone to crying or losing their tempers toward other residents and staff. When vascular dementia is the result of a marked incident, such as a stroke, the loss in function usually plateaus following a period of rehabilitation wherein some abilities may be restored.

## Lewy Body Dementia (LBD)/Parkinsonian Disease Dementia (PDD)

Approximately fifty percent of persons affected by Parkinson's disease develop Lewy body dementia, caused by particles in the brain tissue known as Lewy bodies. Symptoms of LBD/PDD include fluctuations in alertness and attention span, low energy level, staring for extended periods, a blank facial expression, and slower movement.

I knew a man with Parkinsonian dementia who was able to play a good game of chess with me. At times he would confuse the king and queen or land a piece in the wrong square. However, his tactics and strategy were clearly retained. Some days he was slower, and sometimes he would unintentionally knock pieces over, due to typical Parkinsonian large muscle spastic movement.

## Alcohol Dementia

Depending on the degree of brain damage, alcohol dementia can be reversible. I have witnessed the recovery of several residents in skilled nursing facilities with a diagnosis of alcohol dementia. They were forgetful, confused and physically compromised upon admission. After a period of sobriety, proper nutrition, and appropriate sleep routines, they were fully remented.

Other irreversible dementias found in long-term care settings include, but are not limited to:

- Frontal-temporal lobe dementia
- Normal pressure hydrocephalus
- Creutzfeldt-Jakob disease
- Huntington's disease
- HIV/AIDS related dementia: AIDS dementia complex
- Closed head injury

While these forms of dementia are not directly addressed in this book, the principles of person-centered caregiving are just as applicable.

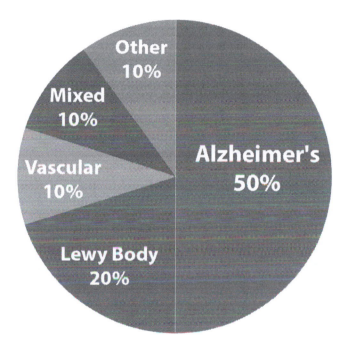

**Figure 1.4** Dementia by Percentages

Readers interested in learning more about dementia are encouraged to research and learn. There are websites and support organizations for each of the conditions above, such as the Alzheimer's Association, American Parkinson's Disease Association, the Huntington's disease Society of America, and so forth. The more caregivers learn, the better we are able to understand the relevance of the care we provide.

## Delirium, Depression, Dementia

Delirium is a temporary condition of dementia-like symptoms. Causes of delirium include but are not limited to infection, dehydration, medication side effects, blood sugar levels and malnutrition. When the factors are addressed with appropriate measures, such as anti-biotic or intravenous therapy, the symptoms of delirium should end within a short period of time.

Many years ago, when I was the receptionist at a law firm with a large window on ground level, I saw a woman in the yard across the street acting oddly. She wore pants with only a brazier on her torso and was crawling on the ground. One of the attorneys came with me to investigate. The woman had lost her glasses and was searching for them. Her speech was slurred, and she was disoriented. At first we assumed she was drunk, though she did not smell of alcohol. She had difficulty walking, yet somehow we brought her back to our office. She told us she was diabetic, homeless, and hungry. We gave her food, drink, and a top to wear. Within 10 minutes or so, she was making sensible conversation and appeared normal. This story is a great example of delirium and how someone can be mistaken as "out of her mind" when the solution to the behavior may be simple.

In long-term care, we often see delirium due to urinary tract infections or dehydration.

The symptoms of dementia and depression can be similar; however, the degree of memory loss is usually greater with dementia. A person with mild to moderate depression should be able to carry out daily tasks when absolutely necessary. Lethargy, characterized by extreme tiredness, can be mistaken for delirium or dementia, but it may be a symptom of severe depression.

Depression is now classified as a mental illness, although Alzheimer's disease and other forms of dementia are not. The signs of depression are caused by *chemical changes* in the brain. Whether caused by a gradual disease process or an acute incident such as a stroke or impact injury, dementia is a result of *physical damage* in the brain. Persons with dementia often have depression. Therefore, proper diagnosis and treatment of depression in the elderly is critical to form a solid plan of care.

To succeed with dementia techniques, we must consider all conditions contributing to a person's limitations, actions, and attitude. Failure to adequately identify and treat depression can result in the patient's loss of appetite, which could then lead to malnutrition and dehydration producing a state of delirium. Staff at long-term care facilities should be trained in reporting the signs and symptoms of depression—a serious illness that affects many aspects of well being.

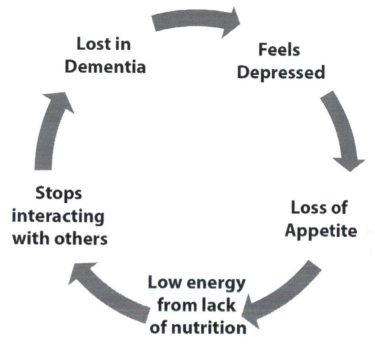

**Figure 1.5** The Depression Cycle

Loss of interest in living, also known as failure to thrive, can be a sign of depression. The condition of dementia itself does not cause depression. Rather, the *change in life circumstances* is what causes depression. Rementia care is good care that supports an individual in living fully with a "now normal," establishing a new level of interaction acceptable for each individual. We can halt the cycle of dementia leading to depression leading to the death of spirit. Read on.

## From Dementia to Rementia

How do we support a shift from a place of not knowing to a place of familiar being? WE BEGIN BY TRANSFORMING THE WAY WE PERCEIVE A PERSON WITH DEMENTIA. We dissolve unfair judgments we have held about limitations and open space for possibilities. As caregivers, we make a commitment to bring our services to the highest level of quality through PERSON-CENTERED CARE philosophy and implementation.

According to Dr. Kitwood, when person-centered care is practiced these are the results:

1. Positive feelings are strengthened.
2. Abilities are nurtured.
3. Psychic wounds are healed.

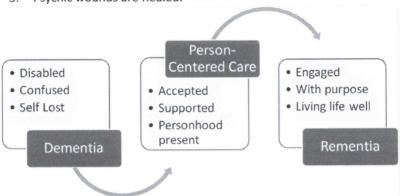

**Figure 1.6** The Path to Rementia

What about the resident who is so consumed by grief he lacks the motivation to rise above his limitations? Certainly all caregivers have encountered this deep sadness. In a few cases, my approaches had little impact. But I never give up trying.

We build the bridge over troubled waters by showing our concern, gaining trust, and respecting each person as worthwhile. Through interpersonal relationships, we save our residents from drowning in dementia. To bond, we cannot fear dementia, be afraid of the unknown, or stay distant because we do not want to be hurt.

"The principal problem, then, is not that of changing people with dementia, or of 'managing' their behavior; it is that of moving beyond our own anxieties and defenses, so that true meeting can occur, and life-giving relationships can grow." (Dr. Kitwood 14)

To make the biggest difference in these delicate lives, we cannot stay in an emotional safety zone. We stretch ourselves further to close the distance between 'us and them.' Compassion is a life vest made of love.

## Validation

Almost every day in the middle of the afternoon, Velma became anxious and would begin asking about her car. Furthermore, she would be attempting to leave the secure unit to find her car because she needed to pick up the kids from school. No amount of distraction could get her mind off this mission. When a caregiver would attempt to divert her attention by offering her a drink or snack, she would say she was too upset to eat or drink. If it was suggested she go to the dining room to join a group activity, she would become more bothered.

*"I can't do that right now. I have to get out of here!"*

*"Velma, what seems to be the problem?"*

*"I'm upset because these people won't help me get out of here. I have to pick up the kids from school, and I need to find my car. I think it's in the parking lot, but I can't get to it. Can you get me out of here?"*

*"Velma, I see you are really worried about the kids. I bet someone else is picking up them up today. Your family knows you are here right now."*

*"Well, I don't know who would pick them up. I do it every day."*

*"Today is different, Velma. For today, you are here, so you don't have to pick them up. I know this is a big change for you. You are such a responsible mother, and you have always done everything for your family. I admire your dedication."*

*"Well, thank you. But now I've got to go, so just show me how to get out of here."*

*"Velma, I really wish there were more I could do for you at this moment. I can't leave right now. And no one else can leave right now either."*

*"What do you mean? Am I in prison? This is a prison and you're keeping me here."*

*"This may seem like a prison because we won't open the door for you to leave, but this is not a prison. I am truly sorry for this trouble. Let's call your son and find out about the kids."*

Then we would call one of her sons, and the son would tell her the kids were fine. I would love to say the trouble ended there, but that was not always the case. Five minutes after calling, Velma would return to my office and start the conversation again, not remembering we had called her son. I would then let her know I had heard from her son that the kids were all right.

After going through the cycle a few times, Velma would become tired and sit down to rest. Often she was in need of a nap, exhausted by her own anxiety. I would see her nodding off in the lobby chair shortly after the episode. The communication was effective because her worries were acknowledged, and she saw me trying to help. Occasions such as these are trying times for caregivers and residents both. To practice person-centered care, we must take the time to respond with concern for well being.

Too many times caregivers deny a resident's self-expression, either ignoring or sometimes trying to convince the resident she is wrong. Arguing leads to an upset resident who may forcefully exit because she feels no one cares. She must leave to find someone who will listen to her plight. Refusing to take the time to listen is poor caregiving. Personal support involves understanding the reality of the other person's despair, despite the facts.

We are *caregivers*, not *care deniers*. Acknowledging another's feelings, without judging right or wrong, is called *validation*. All people need to be validated. If caregivers allow a safe space for residents to express fears and sadness openly and honestly, we can guide them from a state of despair to a peaceful place.

Naomi Feil, author of "The Validation Breakthrough" presented validation therapy as an innovative way to communicate with those suffering from dementia. Her approach begins with viewing the emotional state of a person as real, regardless of the reasons for the emotions. Prior to the practice of Feil's philosophy, reality orientation (RO) was taught as the way to communicate with all residents, with or without dementia, in long-term care settings. The facts of reality can be devastating to a resident who is searching for his wife who passed away years ago. Talking about the facts almost never works out well in that type of situation. Feil's validation therapy advises caregivers to recognize the person's fear or anger or sadness *as reality for that person at that moment* and to find ways to comfort—NOT TO TALK HIM OUT OF FEELINGS BY TELLING HIM THE TRUTH.

Wikipedia (web) summarizes Feil's validation therapy as follows:

> The basic principle of the therapy is the concept of validation or the reciprocated communication of respect which communicates that the other's opinions are acknowledged, respected, heard, and (regardless of whether or not the listener actually agrees with the content), they are being treated with genuine respect as a legitimate expression of their feelings, rather than marginalized or dismissed.

Although validating a person's feelings may not always fix a problem, using lies to settle emotions is not advised. Saying, "Your wife will be here in a little while," when the wife rarely comes to visit is unfair and misleading. Those little white lies can create big trust issues.

> *The heart of the matter is acknowledging the reality of a person's emotions and feelings, and giving a response on the feeling level. Validation involves a high degree of empathy, attempting to understand a person's entire frame of reference, even if it is chaotic or paranoid, or filled with hallucinations. When our experience is validated we feel more alive, more connected, and more real; there is every ground for supposing that this is true in dementia as well. (Dr. Kitwood 91)*

This book is not about throwing out everything we have been doing by calling it all wrong. *Getting REAL About Alzheimer's* is about tilting our heads to see under, over, and around obstacles. In doing so, we can discover what we have never seen before. Are you ready to change the view of caregivers, including your own, in long-term care? If your answer is yes, together we can explore the possibilities. What amazing changes we can work toward practicing rementia care!

## Going Deeper—The Science Behind Dementia and Rementia

Here are a few helpful definitions to get through this next part:

**Neuron or neurones**—brain cells (Neuron is the English spelling, neurones is the British. Dr. Kitwood was British)

**Plaques and tangles**—forms of amyloidal protein build up in the brain

**Neurological**—having to do with brain function

**Synapses**—nerve endings in the brain that transmit information to each other

Do we have control over our own minds? What about the minds of others? Do our brains control our minds? Why don't we use the expression "You're out of your brain?"

I make the decision to drink a cup of coffee to perk me up. Brain studies show the caffeine activates part of the brain and improves ability to concentrate. I had the idea to drink the coffee, which is a thought, widely considered a production of the mind. The decision (have coffee) based on the thought had an effect in my brain (from the caffeine), which then effected my mind (more alert) resulting in a higher productivity. The question of whether or not the mind is contained within the brain has no right answer. However, many people would agree that without a physical brain, the mind does not exist.

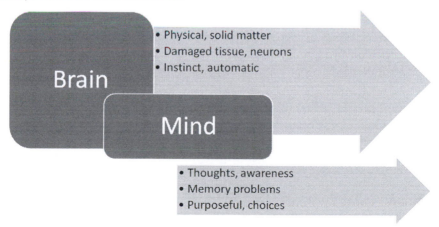

Figure 1.7 Seen and Unseen

> "Now, the brain events or states occur within an 'apparatus' that has a structure, architecture. The key functioning part is a system of around ten thousand million…neurones [British spelling] with their myriads of branches and connections, or synapses. A synapse is the point at which a 'message' can pass from one neurone to another…" (Dr. Kitwood 18)

The responsibility of neurons goes far beyond sending basic messages that tell us how to eat, walk, and talk. Neurons also deliver information about our emotions. This book is about emotional well-being along with survival needs. I am not going into detail about our amazing and complex **brains.** At a minimum, caregivers who practice *rementia* should know that neurons are programmed to do what they do. Babies are not born knowing how to speak. Neurons are 'trained,' thus we learn to speak.

Different sections of the brain are responsible for memory, mood, large body movement, the five senses of sound, smell, taste, touch, vision, automatic functions (such as breathing and heartbeat), mood, and many, many, other functions. Remembering what our senses tell us about what they perceive (smell food cooking, going to eat soon) is just the beginning of a lifetime of learning. Our brains are developing as we learn and grow. Perhaps the process only stops when we lose our interest in learning or cease to be intellectually challenged.

In the process of AD, formations of amyloidal protein called plaques and tangles interfere with neuron communication. These plaques and tangles prevent information from being sent from one nerve ending to another. A signal is sent for the word "food" but is blocked between neurons, so the word does not come out of the person's mouth or comes out as a different word.

Current theory is that neurons die when they are not able to complete transmissions. Thus, in a brain affected by AD, there is a considerable amount of dead brain tissue. The average healthy brain weighs 3 lbs. However, the brain of a person who dies from AD weighs significantly less. For a good view of the brain and its inner workings, visit www.alz.org.

## Transforming How We Give Care

This book is about transformation. Some of the ideas may seem like common sense. Others may seem too far "out there." *Getting REAL* is for caregivers who want a brighter future for those with dementia and who want to be a direct part of seeing the results of practicing person-centered care. Transformation begins with accepting a theory, considering possibilities, and committing to take steps to promote change.

Throughout this book, we are going to explore healing in numerous ways. The concept of caregivers—with any level of education and training—serving as emotional healers should be welcomed. Without having a license to perform surgery or prescribe medication or give professional counseling, we can be healers by incorporating a sense of honor in the services we provide. We can practice person-centered care and believe in the power of rementia to create new neurological functioning in the brain of persons with Alzheimer's and all types of dementia.

After delivering twins, one of my best friends developed a blood clot in her brain. After it burst, her brain swelled (hydrocephalus) to twice its normal size. To accommodate the size, a piece of her skull was removed and kept alive under a skin flap in her abdomen until the brain returned to normal size. Then, like a lid, the piece of skull was put back in place. What a procedure! Due to the cerebral vascular accident (CVA), Caroline was paralyzed on one side of her body for weeks. She could barely speak for months, and she could not read or write for a few years.

Today, Caroline can drive, cook dinner, pay her bills, slowly read and write, and have conversations with some delay finding the right words. Though she still has a degree of short term and long term memory loss, with each year she improves, and she can retrieve information when prompted with the right clues. Her family and friends were invested in her recovery, and she was surrounded by people who loved her while healing. She had skilled therapists, too. Physical, occupational, and speech therapists play a major role in *rementing* stroke patients. Unfortunately, people with dementia often receive limited therapies because measurable progress—harder to achieve with cognitive impairment—must be shown within a certain time frame.

How did Caroline recover? Can the same happen with forms of dementia if we invest extended time and patience? If we lose faith in people with brain conditions and do not challenge them to function and interact at the highest possible level, the chances of rementia are slim.

How does a resident with middle stage AD learn her way to the dining room when she enters a new place of living? Some never do and require daily reminders. Yet many do learn their way around independently. We do not have to know whether information is encoded through old neurons, repaired neurons, new neurons or previously unused neurons. We need to have faith that persons with dementia can experience new growth and personal development.

Dr. Kitwood states that "...social psychology works to offset the process of neurological decline." (Dr. Kitwood 5)

In the United States, social psychology is more commonly known as "psychosocial." Section 2, "Engagement," focuses on the importance of meeting psychosocial needs. An environment in which residents thrive creates positive changes in the mind and in the brain itself. We must act to promote the concept that meaningful engagement, appropriate levels of assistance, and a loving workplace atmosphere lead to fulfillment for the entire population. Caregivers can contribute to dysfunction, or use rementia methods to become healers.

Rementia theory is not about *curing* AD. The degenerative process of the brain disease is not likely to stop because Mr. Williams is stimulated spending time in the garden. However, his life has been of a much higher quality since his mind/brain/spirit found a way to live as a whole person again. In summary:

**Dementia** is about "HE CANNOT!"

**Rementia** is about "HE CAN!"

What are we waiting for?

# TILT Keys on Rementia

1. What do you think of the term "healer?"

2. Did you feel influenced at any point reading this section? If so, when and why?

3. Have you ever witnessed a case of rementia? Tell the story.

4. What staff practices have you seen that contribute to resident decline?

5. On a scale of 1-5, with 5 as total understanding, how well do you get the meaning of *rementia*?

    1    2    3    4    5

6. Please rate the following statement:

   *Without increasing the number of staff on each shift, transformation can occur through person-centered care practices.*

Strongly Agree    Agree    Not Sure    Disagree    Strongly Disagree

7. Which statement describes your opinion about using validation for emotional support? (You can check more than one)

_____ I believe validation can and should be practiced at all times.

_____ I am not sure I understand how to use validation.

_____ I would like to try it, but there just is not enough time in the day.

_____ Sometimes I use validation and it works to comfort residents.

_____ I feel like validation is a form of not telling the truth.

8. Name three person-centered care approaches you already use.

9. What do you feel is good about the service you provide?

10. Circle the words that describe how you feel about persons with dementia:

Hopeful Sad Afraid Positive Confused Uncertain Educated Frustrated Understanding Confident

# Section 2: Engagement

## Engagement—Creating a Whole New World

A daughter comes to tour a care community because she feels the family can no longer assure her mother is safe and healthy at home. The daughter is looking for the best facility and is very concerned her mother will not like any place other than home. Her mother no longer sees the need to change into clean clothes or shower.

I have never known the marketing representative to say, "Well, tell you what. Bring your mom over for a visit. We'll start by giving her a shower to see if she likes us!"

In reality, what we recommend is the daughter and the mom come for a group activity, such as a musical performance or party. Maybe we suggest they sit in the garden and have a cup of coffee or come for lunch, and to meet a few other ladies. We are putting the **engagement** experience first. Shouldn't we continue on that path even after the mother is admitted? Yes, and that is why we must make time for person-centered engagement along with the other duties we make a priority before the end of the day. Social needs and physical well-being go hand in hand.

> **engage**—*v*. To attract and hold: *a project that engaged her interest*. To participate: *engage in conversation*. (*The American Heritage*)
> **engaged**—*adj*. Employed, occupied, or busy. (*The American Heritage*)

In the past, physical needs have been regarded as more important than psychosocial needs. When it comes to life or death, this is the case. However, lack of a person-centered approach can contribute to depression, which can contribute to physical decline and lead to premature death. As caregivers become enlightened, the possibility of healing through engagement grows stronger.

> **transform**—v. To change in structure, appearance or character (*Merriam Webster*)
>
> **transform**—v. To change in nature or condition (*The American Heritage*)

Our earlier discussion in Section 1 stated that *Getting REAL* is about **transformation**: we are altering the structure and character of how to meet the needs of our residents to promote **rementia**. The primary component of rementia is **engagement**, also *known as* **activities**. True engagement occurs when we begin practicing **person-centered care.** Though these ideas seem to be obvious, they are not so simple. To change the structure of how we provide services is a big deal. Very big and very possible.

To begin, we re-evaluate our own personal beliefs about what is most important on a daily to-do list. Historically, activities have been the responsibility of staff who are trained on how to do certain types of interaction, and only those staff members plan and spend time doing activities. At my last place of service, the job expectation was for personal care assistants to be involved in engagement as much as possible throughout the shift.

Some readers, particularly those who work in skilled nursing/intermediate long-term care facilities (SNF/ICF), may reject this idea. The common conception that assisted living (AL) staff does not have a workload as heavy as those in SNF/ICF settings is not necessarily true. In an Assisted Living Memory Care (ALMC) unit, the staffing ratio is often higher than in the SNF/ICF standards. Although the argument is made that the level of care is heavier in the SNF/ICF, this is not always the case. There can be several bed bound persons on hospice services in an ALMC community. The load on an assigned section in ALMC can be just as heavy as in a SNF/ICF.

A few select individuals in the activities and social service department cannot satisfy all of the *social and personal needs* of a large population. As the overall well being of residents has become a larger issue in recent years, we must find new ways to meet needs beyond keeping a person clean, safe and "fed." **Engagement is an activity of daily living.**

## Go Psychosocial for Your Residents

*Psychosocial needs* are the unseen, often unmet needs of those with Alzheimer's disease and other forms of dementia. A person may not be able to state "There's nothing to do around here" or "Nobody cares. They walk by without saying a word to me." Therefore, we may underestimate the importance of that individual's need or desire to be active in a meaningful or fun manner. Even more likely, there may be episodes labeled as negative "behavior" because a person is feeling restless or disregarded.

> **psychosocial** — combination of the words "psychological" and "social," *psychosocial* needs are about an individual's relationships with others.
> **psychological**—having to do with the mind, related to mental processes. One definition includes "directed toward the will."
> **social—has a variety of meanings, including:**
> "Related to the interaction of people,"
> "The way in which people behave in groups," and even
> "Living as part of a community."

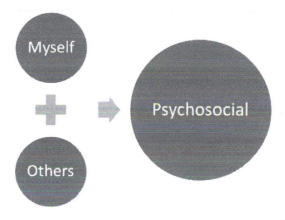

**Figure 2.1** Psychosocial Circles

Psychosocial needs pertain to an individual's view of herself individually and as a part of a group. These needs are harder to identify than physical needs and must be recognized while assisting with the overall care process. Meeting psychosocial needs goes much further than making small talk while we are helping with grooming—though conversation is a great start and makes a difference. Psychological needs include feelings of trust, belonging, acceptance, satisfaction, understanding, respect, and honor.

What if you come into work one day and no one says hello—not at the front desk, not at the time clock, not when you walk into the area where you are assigned. No one looks your way, makes eye contact, or speaks a word to you. What if the only interaction you have is about what task has to be done next. No laughing or smiling or anyone saying "Boy, I am so tired!" or "I'm hungry—I can't wait until lunch!" Just work, work, work. No sense of being accepted by or connected to those around you.

Soon you would begin to feel left out and wonder what is wrong with you. Or perhaps you would become defensive and decide your coworkers are rude. Either way, you would not be comfortable and most likely would not want to go back to that workplace.

When our psychosocial needs are not met, our mental health is adversely affected. We may become withdrawn or angry or confused. Not investing the time to interact on a meaningful level with those we serve is jeopardizing their psychological needs.

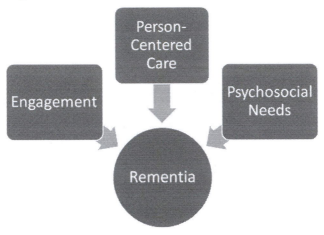

**Figure 2.2** Forming Rementia

Notice in the diagram above there is no mention of meeting the physical needs of those we serve. The main purpose in writing this book is to promote transformation from a model of caregiving wherein emphasis is on physical needs to emphasis placed on the less obvious needs. This concept is not meant to imply food is secondary to having a social life. Food is what keeps our bodies alive, and without good nutrition, no one is going to be having any fun. However, the showers, meals, and incontinent care fall into a natural rhythm when providing person-centered care. If approached with rementia in mind, a caregiver can use Activities of Daily Living (ADL's) to help patients heal more than a physical condition.

## Finding Lost Personhood

Personhood is a term used to describe the individual self. Typically during the admissions process, a questionnaire is completed to learn about new residents. The standard survey is a great start for getting basic information used to determine what type of activities will appeal to a new person.

Within the first few weeks, the program manager or social worker should conduct an extended life interview with residents and families, then place copies in a binder for all staff to read. The variety of life circumstances and rich histories we have around us every day are fascinating. Consider asking questions such as these:

*Where were you born? Did you travel? Were you in the military? What is your strongest childhood memory? Tell me about your family. What's your favorite color? Of what are you most proud? Do you like to be outside? What are your favorite foods? Are you afraid of spiders or snakes? Would you rather watch a movie or read a book? Do you live a spiritual life?*

Although people with AD are not always able to fully answer questions, an interview is great one-on-one time. Responses hold keys to meaningful engagement. Family members and others who know the resident should also be interviewed. I once had a resident tell me he was a farmer. His son told me his father was a hairdresser. The father had no accessible memories of being a hairdresser. He wanted to be outside with his hands in the dirt.

History is only one aspect of personhood. Everybody changes during life, and a man who once played piano may have no interest in playing now or may no longer be able to play. Likewise, someone who did crocheting for many years may no longer have the fine motor skills to do so, and we must find new hobbies or ways to modify the hobby. I once had a women tell me to bug off (except those are not the choice words she used) when I asked if she wanted to help with the cookies. She had her share of domestic activity as a housewife—thank you very much.

If someone were to ask you what you do on your days off, your response would be a good reflection of your personhood. Person-centered engagement is about opening possibilities for how residents spend the hours of each day, now that each day is a day off! To develop activities based on individuality we combine an individual's past and present personhood. We should know important facts about what makes him or her HIM or HER. Find out what triggers pleasure as well as what feelings of fear or discomfort.

When residents are new to a place, they may hardly know who they are anymore. Dementia may rule the person in this strange environment. Caregivers uncover traits of personhood beneath layers of defensiveness, hurt and grief.

This process may or may not take a while. Sometimes a connection is made easily, though we should not expect to waltz into a resident's room and be instant friends. The new setting may cause added confusion for several days or even weeks after admission-the adjustment period varies. A person may not show preferences, want to attend activities or be involved with other residents. However, even the most distant new resident will usually interact during private visits. One-to-one engagement may be required for months, even years.

> *It's only when the care partner really understands the resident-including history, current views and preferences, spirituality and values, and what tends to trigger anger or unhappiness-and gains the person's trust that effective, non-pharmacological interventions can take place. (Lourde 26)*

The author quoted above refers to "non-pharmacological interventions." In long-term care, we are closely exploring how to reduce medications used to decrease agitation. Modern pharmaceuticals used to treat thought and mood disorders can be very helpful in improving quality of life. Yet, I recall the days of over medicating and do not favor returning to medication used as a restraint. To conform with an ever increasing regulatory environment, we must develop creative activity programs. Certain medications will be reduced, as will the number of incident reports written due to the negative "behaviors" resulting from unmet needs. There are no negative side effects from a hearty regimen of engagement.

Promoting personhood despite physical and mental limitations is the cornerstone of a life well lived. Using the questionnaire method to gather personal facts is valuable when building an engagement program. But nothing beats direct observation of how residents interact and react to stimulation when assessing which activities are most beneficial. **By listening and observing we learn what is important to an individual during the present period.** Once explored, the history and current preferences assist staff in guiding residents to activities that match the individual's full picture profile.

**Rementia comes about by exercising skills that are still in place and finding meaningful activities that provide a sense of achievement.** Even if working memory is impaired to the point of inability to follow instructions, residents who become involved in group projects form new social ties with those around them. Some will be "doers" and some will be "watchers." Both will be engaged. However, a resident frustrated during an activity should be offered an alternative way to engage. Otherwise, the activity may go downward for everyone.

Engagement is more than organized activities such as entertainment, exercise and projects. People with dementia benefit greatly from focused one-to-one interaction, and the interaction need not wait until a state of despair is present. Many residents will not attend group activities, large or small, and one-to-one chats or working on a project individually are the only means for self expression. Ah, but still *time is the predicament.*

> *Most people in long-term care like these ideas…but are worried that having caregivers engage in meaningful conversations with residents as they provide care—or merely as they see them in the common areas—would take up so much time that they wouldn't be able to fulfill all the regulatory requirements. (Lourde 30)*

A caregiver may believe it is unrealistic for her to spend time talking about a resident's past or that she cannot take twenty minutes to read a magazine to a group of attentive residents.

> *Just affirm those creative words—next time, can, and possible. And be like every good positive thinker, be a word dropper and throw out if, can't and impossible. (Peale 149)*

Section 3 explores ways to fulfill job duties while meeting the emotional, spiritual, deeper needs of our residents. The first step is the desire to be a healer through powerful engagement. Can we create more time for spontaneous fun and much needed one-to-one heartfelt communication?

By the end of this book, my aim is for the readers' answers to be "**YES, I understand how I can make that happen.**"

## Appropriate Level of Activity

Our goal is to occupy residents in meaningful activities, to encourage leisure time, and to have fun! We do this by focusing on **person-centered care** engagement. The following are good ideas that deserve to be repeated!

> *How do we conduct an engagement program based on person-centered care theory?*

> *Person-centered care acknowledges each person as unique with a unique experience of life. Are you seeing him as a person with unique preferences?*

Would you ever show up unannounced and say to a friend, "Come on, hurry up, and get your shoes on. We're going to a party now!" You wouldn't, because you have a personal relationship with your friends. Friends discuss when and where they are going together. Even a simple, "Hi Nancy, I'm going to the party in the dining room. Would you like to join me?" is an invitation that prompts choice.

At this time the readers may think giving such basic advice is absurd. Is it? Or am I bringing to life a new way of interacting?

Rather than overly trying to convince a person to participate or placing the person in a setting that has no meaning, residents can be encouraged to take part in activities that are based on interaction. For activities to be appropriate, residents should only be taken to group functions where participation is possible. An activity should match an individual's cognitive (mental) and physical abilities.

**A resident who repeatedly asks "what are we doing here?" during an activity is not in the appropriate group.**

If during trivia games a resident never attempts to answer any questions, she may not be in the right level of activity. Likewise, if a resident is unable to hold a paintbrush, she should not be sitting at a table with paints and paper placed in front of her. Is there any visible evidence that residents are engaged?

> *How do we know if we are doing person-centered care engagement?*

> *Person-centered care engagement promotes an individual's highest level of function by applying what is known about that person while services are being provided. Is she interested?*

If a resident is sleeping—not just nodding off, but is actively snoring—for dignity, safety, and comfort reasons guide him to his room or a quiet place.

> *How do we decide who should go to an activity when people with dementia have such varying levels of ability and understanding?*

> *In person-centered care, each person participating is a "meaning-maker" in the source of action. Interaction occurs as each participant interprets the meaning of the others' actions. Watch for signs that residents are stimulated, such as facial expressions, verbal responses, and body language. Does he appreciate the objective of this activity?*

Intentionally, I am not breaking activities into stage levels of AD. No one should be limited based on assumptions. In early stage AD, ability to follow simple instruction is usually intact. In middle stage, working memory (step by step instruction) is usually impaired. However, I have had a woman in early stage unable to cut up celery who kept asking what to do. Yet next to her a woman in middle stage quickly chopped her stalks, arranged them beautifully on the plate, and let me know that removing the stringy fibers makes celery get mushy when cooked. Interest and ability may vary on different days or times of the day. Knowing residents' patterns and baselines is helpful. Often a change in health condition is identified by a change in participation during activities.

Sometimes a staff member will bring a resident to an activity because she is demonstrating a difficult "behavior." Sometimes this redirection may work. Sometimes it causes a bigger problem. Before relying on a group activity as the answer, be sure there is not a basic need or health condition to address. Is she hungry, angry, tired or in need of "freshening up?"

> *It is essential that the administrator not permit the activities program to be turned into a glorified babysitting service. (Buettner, Legg 48)*

Leaving a person lying in a geri-chair for exercise class is using the activity room as a parking lot. Again, activities should be selected based on a resident's capabilities and personal interest. I have seen far too many activity calendars with once a day one-size-fits-all exercise class. **Rarely is any activity a one-size-fits-all.** A good activities program is based on true engagement, wherein each participant is getting something out of the interaction.

These questions can guide decisions regarding participation level of individuals:

> *How much working memory is required to do this task?*
> *Is the participant free to move at a natural pace?*
> *If unable to follow step by step direction, is the activity enjoyable or frustrating to watch as an observer?*

In intermediate/skilled nursing facilities funded by Medicare and Medicaid, the Federal standard of operation regulation F-248 states:

> *"The facility involves the resident in an ongoing program of activities that is designed to appeal to his or her interests and to enhance the resident's highest practicable level of physical, mental, and psychological well-being." (CMS, web)*

**Sounds like person-centered care!**

At my last position as program manager for memory care services, I started modified yoga classes. As a person who has practiced yoga for many years, I believe in the benefits of this mental, spiritual and physical exercise. Professional and highly skilled yoga instructors were willing to lend their expertise at a reduced hourly rate because they know the benefits of yoga for persons of all ages and abilities.

For the class to be of maximum benefit, I experimented with multiple participants to see how they responded. Some did not want to sit long enough and would leave, a few would talk out loud too much during class, a few would fall asleep, one would just stare at the instructor, and one was frustrated to the point of tears by her physical limitations (a symptom of vascular dementia due to stroke.) Each week, I would substitute new members for those who were unable to stay put and follow instructions. A blend of 13 became the regular attendees, a perfect size for a yoga class.

Katherine Sasseen, one of the instructors, says of this group:

> The memory care patients seem to respond to yoga. The participants do the best they can within their physical limits. As we progress through the breathing exercises and modified chair asanas, I notice shifts physically and energetically. Some may need to clear their throats or cough a little bit because the energy begins to flow and is released, and they let go. The neck relaxes and the throat opens. They breathe deeper and relax. Posture also improves. The spine lengthens. Body, mind, and spirit let go of restrictions. This sometimes causes reactions like giggling and humming along with the music. They get into their own rhythm of breathing and moving. Some have eyes open. Some have eyes closed. I ask them to notice how they are feeling at This Moment. We have a gratitude practice. After class, everyone applauds and says thank you.
>
> The women appear on the whole to not be agitated, even if they had been prior to yoga practice. Some ask questions after class. A few hug me or reach out and hold my hand. One day as I was leaving, a woman who was sitting in a large armchair who hadn't participated much physically stopped me and said "I really enjoyed that. I didn't really do much of it but I really felt it. It was beautiful!"

Yoga class is an example of person centered engagement and the importance of leveling members based on interest and capability. Even the woman quoted in the last paragraph got something out of the class with her physical limitations. Class is set in the middle of the afternoon, which works very well for those who are not morning people and never make it to the morning exercise class. Opportunities to exercise throughout the day should be part of the programming to meet the needs of different body rhythms.

Because 13 in the yoga class are only 20 percent of the resident population, other opportunities for engagement must be happening simultaneously. Because the class is held by an outside instructor, the lifestyle assistant who conducts calendared events is free to orchestrate other activities during class time.

## Yoga and More Rementia Story

 Carolyn, the instructor, was relieved when she recognized Joyce in yoga class. Joyce was a former student of Carolyn's from a local yoga studio prior to Joyce's transition to assisted living. Although Joyce did not remember Carolyn or the yoga studio, she did recall having a yoga practice. A member of class each week, Joyce demonstrates her retained knowledge of familiar movements from her yoga practice. And there is more to the story of Joyce.

Prior to her admittance to the facility where I worked, Joyce had resided in another assisted living memory care establishment. She had not been happy there, so the family had moved her. The staff at the prior community said Joyce had "behavior" such as aggressiveness toward staff and frequently entering the rooms of other residents uninvited.

When we reviewed her history during a manager's meeting, I declared she would not have such difficulty with us. We would keep her engaged. And so it is.

Joyce has free will to go outside—the previous memory care unit is located on the second floor—and Joyce is an outdoor person fond of gardening. She now has her yoga practice and good relationships with others. There have been no incidences involving aggressive behavior or other resident's rooms. One yoga instructor states that Joyce often says to her "They do a pretty good job around here, don't you think?"

**From difficult "behavior" to meaningful living. That's transformation. The case for the power of rementia is growing stronger.**

## Components of Structured Engagement

### The Calendar of Scheduled Events

Many residents want to know what is happening each day and rely on the calendar to see what social opportunities are planned. A comprehensive calendar is the pillar in a well structured program. There are many websites, such as www.activityconnection.com, that are resources for designing calendars and finding ideas for new and different activities. There are also many books written by experts in the field of long-term care recreation that can be used as guides for creating outstanding programs.

Consultant Nancy Schier Anzelmo of Alzheimer's Care Associates LLC, recommends calendars designed with blocks of activities throughout the day with definitive break times between blocks for ADL assistance. I used her suggestion and had activities in the main room starting at 9:00 a.m. and ending at 11:00 a.m., then starting back up at 1:00 p.m., and ending again at 4:00 p.m. An evening block was from 6:00 p.m. to 8:00 p.m. A schedule with this format allows time for residents before and after meals to "freshen up." When I first put this system in place, the care assistants exclaimed,

"What about those who don't need to freshen up? What are they supposed to do for 45 minutes before lunch?"

The lifestyle assistant, or activity director, can still be available to do small group or one to one engagement in the dining room as residents trickle in from other areas.

When a calendar is set up with activities one after the other right up until lunch time, a "herd-like" appearance tends to form as the group is led to the dining room all together, often in a hurried fashion because the activity ended five minutes before the meal service. Again, buffer time between activities and meals is needed for a more natural flow.

## Large Group Events

Big events are big engagement times. As stated earlier, residents should give their consent before going to an activity. Look for non-verbal cues to see if the resident is enjoying the activity. When taken into a room with people doing exercise, does the resident smile or shake her head in a "no" manner?

A few best practices for large group events, such as musical performances and parties:

- Be sure to have seating arranged so there are clear pathways to doors.
- Do not block pathways with wheelchairs or walkers.
- Non-ambulatory persons should be seated at the ends of rows where the pathways are located, thus in an emergency they can be removed first or if they need assistance during an event the entire row will not be disturbed.
- Persons who are known to have a history of incompatibility should be seated as far away from each other as possible.
- Persons who are known to get up and leave during a performance or who have frequent needs to "freshen up" should be seated at the ends of rows and nearest to exit doors.
- An overcrowded room could present major problems during an emergency—be sure the amount of persons at an event would allow for smooth evacuation.
- Stay mindful of the territorial issues that arise when the dining room is used for engagement other than meals. Seating a person at a table where another person is accustomed to sitting for meals can cause a disturbance.

Participation in large group events is a healthy way for individuals to feel belonging and connection to others. Parties are great ways to celebrate life, and I have had more fun dancing and singing with residents at care communities than at parties outside of care communities. Staff members should encourage residents to express themselves (appropriately!) and encourage each other to express themselves (appropriately!) to make parties true to life.

***Let go during parties! Have some fun! Dance like no one is watching!***

The most dismal sight is walking into a dining room where the "party" is happening and residents are not responding to the musical guest or slumped over asleep in their chairs. Group events are "activities" during which there should be signs of life! CELEBRATE WITH THOSE YOU SERVE! CELEBRATE YOURSELF! CELEBRATE PERSONHOOD!

> *Many people who have dementia, despite their suffering, retain the capacity to celebrate; perhaps it is even enhanced as the burdens of responsibility disappear. Celebration is the form of interaction in which the division between caregiver and cared-for comes nearest to vanishing completely; all are taken up into a similar mood. (Dr. Kitwood 90-91)*

During the progression of dementia, some areas in the right side of the brain are preserved longer than in the left side. Creativity, like artistic traits, comes from the right side of the brain, as do language skills and automatic language (that explains the swearing!) No wonder almost 100% of residents in long-term care settings respond so well to music and dance.

Large groups, however, are not for everyone during every phase of living. Some people have never been much for crowds. No one should be stuck and unable to leave a group activity, and if there are signs of discomfort from those who cannot get up and walk out, respond to the need before the whole audience is affected.

> *If the activity is disturbed by the presence of residents who are inappropriate for the activity, it is likely that the residents' enjoyment will be low... (Buettner, Legg 48)*

## Small Group Engagement

We all have personal forms of relaxing, communicating, and expression; thus residents respond differently to types of stimulation. Small group projects are to target skills of a group who have similar interests. The modular system presented later in this section is a tool for successful small groups.

Small group activities are interactive, based on a common goal (fixing a snack) or shared desire for companionship (talking during tea time) or social structure (playing games). *In small groups, it should be obvious whether or not participants get something out of attending. No one should be just occupying a chair or sleeping. Taking a quick nap in the sunshine is one thing—snoring during bingo is another!* Small groups allow self-expression and the opportunity for individual residents to be of assistance to others, a great way to promote self-esteem.

> *If a resident shows an "inability to effectively function in a group activity setting, then individualized activities to meet [her] unique needs should be developed." (Buettner, Legg 48)*

For example, during a small art class of five persons, one woman is sitting at a table with watercolors. Although she can still hold the brush, her working memory (following step by step procedures) has faded. Her face is as blank as the sheet of paper put before her. Across the table, another woman is asking "What do you want me to do?" The activity leader is helping a man hold a brush and making strokes for him saying "Oooh that looks pretty!" Perhaps there are two participants at the table who are engaged by painting independently. Three persons are not participating effectively. An alternative form of stimulation should be presented, such as looking at a book of paintings while the two who can paint continue. A little sing-along or storytelling can add to the activity. **USE YOUR IMAGINATION TO BE AN ENGAGEMENT STAR!**

Here's another non-engagement scenario with a holiday card making activity. Only a few of the participants are ***making the cards*** as the activity leader is cutting paper (*can't let them use scissors, too dangerous*), applying the glue (*can't let them use the glue—that's messy!*), then sprinkling on the glitter (*might get it in their eyes!*). What we really have going on: activities are being 'done to' the people. Many of the residents could probably care less about the outcome because they have invested nothing from their own abilities in the process.

**Rementia is promoted when residents contribute.**

If Dr. Kitwood's theory is true—that not using the mind contributes to the decline in mental function—would those of us caring for people with dementia ensure minds are stimulated every day? What if you could see neurons dying inside a person's brain as she absently stares off into the distance during the above activity? Would you continue the project as it was? What if every time a resident was "getting something" out of an activity you could see neurons inside of the brain lighting up as they fired information back and forth? Would you be inclined to lead more appropriate level activities?

If you could physically see the neurons being activated while you promoted engagement, you would know you are a healer. **Know you are**

**a healer even without that kind of visible proof.** Know you are a healer every time you hear a resident say, "I did it!"

# Obstacles To Engagement

As discussed earlier, limited time is the number one reason there is not enough engagement in long-term care settings. In the next section on Assistance, we are going to explore how providing activities of daily living can be more interactive. Right now, I want to propose some underlying reasons for the lack of engagement throughout the day.

Barriers to transforming recreation programs include:

**Fear**—might put residents at risk, have an accident with injury
Solution—discuss your concerns with others, get feedback on safety, and try the activity at the lowest level of risk before increasing exposure. If your fear is based on a past incident, review the circumstances and eliminate any conditions that are within your control. Realize that accidents happen even when we are doing our best.

**Empty Excuses**—need to call boyfriend, smoke a cigarette, finish coffee, gossip
Solution—Honor your agreement to your place of employment and those you serve. Re-commit to engagement. No sneaking away or hiding out. Follow the employee code of conduct by limiting personal business to break times. Spending too much time on the clock talking about non-work related matters is a violation against your residents.

**Being Human**—feeling tired, having a bad day, no creative flow
Solution—Everyone has a bad day now and then. Let your supervisor know when you are not at your best. Ask for understanding and a little extra time to rest between big tasks. Ask for support from co-workers. Let them know you will make it up somehow when you feel up to par. Then keep your word and go the extra mile next time.

**Lack of Confidence**—don't know what to do, out of ideas, not good at activities, embarrassed, shy
Solution—Residents with dementia are the most forgiving audience of all. Just about anything goes for entertainment. Experiment until you find what feels natural. Let go of your doubts and let your inner light shine. You'll be glad you did.

**Inconvenience**—too much trouble, makes a mess, not in the mood
Solution—Activities can be messy and require extra effort. Being a caregiver for those with AD is not convenient work and may not be for you.

Some of the reasons that limit the commitment to engagement are valid. Once we see the value in person-centered care, we find ways to go beyond a belief system of limitations. Those of us who believe in rementia are on board for an adventure that leads everyone to good living and maximum health. The following information is about a system that supports both residents and staff members to be successful at activities.

# User-Friendly Organized Systems

A modular system is a stock of supplies organized by themes and accessible for all staff to begin engagement WHEREVER and WHENEVER needed. Late afternoon when the structured calendar has a break between large group afternoon activities and dinner, the modules are a handy source for unplanned fun and involvement. Design your own modules or follow the categories outlined below. Create what works for your unique population.

## Modules

Modules are best organized in clear plastic storage bins of varying sizes. Use smaller, portable containers for mobility. Keep supplies in multiple containers stored in a variety of locations. White mailing labels work well for keeping supplies in the right containers. When shopping for games and puzzles, keep in mind the size of the box and buy large plastic baggies to store pieces after the boxes have been ruined. Be sure to cut out the small photo of the puzzle from the box to keep in the bag with the pieces. Large sealed baggies are also a must for many art supplies and food preparation items.

A reasonable budget for purchasing a good number of storage bins and starter supplies is $150-200. During initial training, all new caregivers are oriented by the program manager or activity director on the module system. This is how mine was set up:

1. Games—puzzles (50 to 100 pieces, inch sized), standard card decks, dice, trivia decks, bingo (I say give them what they want, but not all day every day!), charades, checkers, etc...
2. Outdoor recreation—blow bubbles, play badminton (not kidding), lightweight ball, play music, a sing along, have refreshments, read from a book or pass around magazines, do stretches, set up a putting green (this is hours of fun inside, too)

3.  Hobbies—flower arranging (change out vases for each season or month), holiday decorations, watercolors, colored pencils and scrap paper, card making, yarn sorting, jewelry making with extra large beads and hemp

4.  Food Prep—always have plastic gloves in module for residents and staff. No exceptions. Make sandwiches (PBJ, sliced cheese), crackers with PB or pimento cheese and liverwurst spread, bake cookies in toaster oven and frost and decorate, sort beans, shred or chop lettuce or celery (plastic knife will work), roll dough, fruit salad, smoothies (easy to cut & peel fruits), vegetable soup (in crock pot). Toaster oven, crock pot and blender—all you need for a makeshift kitchen. For infection control purposes, residents cannot eat while preparing though they can when all is ready! Allow participants to clean up afterwards, too. That's Module 10.

5.  Music—print out lyrics from old songs and make songbooks, use maracas, tambourines, bells, woodwind instruments, (all are noisy and so much fun!) ask a resident who plays piano to perform, ask management for permission to use your cellular device to play age appropriate music.

6.  SPA—lightly scented hand lotions, petroleum jelly for lips (apply with Q-tips), manicure supplies (disposable nail files, round ended wooden sticks for cleaning under nails.) Residents can file their own nails if able and unless prohibited by facility policy, regulations and/or medical conditions, caregivers can clip nails, do cleaning, and paint nails. If there is no appropriate public area to use as a spa, ask ladies to volunteer their own rooms to gather. Spa activities may vary greatly according to regulations.

7.  Exercise—chair exercise DVDs or lead class with music, balloon toss (always a fun success for a wide range of ability), yoga, stretch bands, dancing to music (always fun!), jog in place, jumping jacks (old-school stuff).

8.  In Community—go on walks around community grounds and, if permissible, in immediate neighborhood, outings, scenic drives. If residents live in a secured area, attend events in the open assisted living area.

9.  Literature/Storytelling—newspaper (keep it positive), magazines, Reader's Digest condensed story collections, inspirational books, religious texts, photo albums, history pictorials. Read out loud or ask a resident to volunteer. Residents really enjoy listening to a steady voice telling a story. Share personal stories back and forth. Starting a simple conversation can lead to hearing great stories.

10. Around the House—keep rags for residents' domestic urges and let them wipe down the dining room chairs or sweep the floor—this is helpful! No chemicals are needed. Any aged person will tell you hot soapy water works best. Keep a laundry basket of lost and found clothing (wash cloths and socks are great but anything will do) for folding. Then bundle them up and store for next time! Keep a big jar of buttons for sorting into colors or sizes (obviously not for anyone with an advanced form of dementia who may put them in her mouth).

A module system makes it easy to match staff talents with appropriate levels of activity for residents in small groups.

- Some people do best in large groups (10 + participants during activity room exercise, game player's choice, musical guests, parties)
- Some people are more successful in smaller groups (3-9 participants doing arts & crafts, playing a dice game, playing balloon volleyball—one of my favorites!)
- Some people prefer solitude with individual activity (putting together a puzzle alone, reading a magazine, sitting out by the fish pond alone) and
- Some people may only respond to one on one communication (viewing photos together, getting nails done, conversation, etc...)
- Some people like it all!

## Activity Aprons

Staff on my last project wore half aprons as part of the uniform. They were perfect for activities on the go. By carrying a few small items in one of the apron pockets, quick engagement can be accomplished anywhere. Suggestions are two balloons, a deck of cards or a few trivia cards from any guessing game, five dice, and a travel size container of lotion.

# Enriching Lives

I hope this section leaves a firm impression on the necessity of engagement. Creating even the smallest moments of connectivity makes for a better day. Somewhere in time, perhaps we will find methods to do it all without hesitation, reluctance and time constraints. In the meantime, the hokey-pokey can be done anywhere, anytime and in five minutes. Just imagine those neurons dancing along, too.

> *Despite the decreased mental and physical functions associated with dementia, it is possible to create an environment in which both a person's physical and psychosocial needs are met, where they feel valued and respected and where they are treated the way they want to be treated. That is exactly what person-centered dementia care accomplishes. (Tucker 45)*

Person centered engagement is about having choices for how to participate in daily living. Personhood is respected as a resident is free to express preferences and personality. The way to rementia is counting on caregivers who are actively involved with the persons in their care and willing to take chances. In the end—after learning from our mistakes—we celebrate ourselves for twisting and turning and tripping and trying again and again until we get the magic right.

As a popular slogan says, "What if the hokey pokey really is what it's all about?"

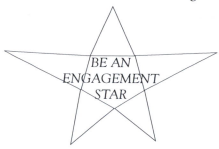

# TILT Keys on Engagement

1. What SKILLS AND TALENTS DO YOU HAVE to be an ENGAGEMENT STAR?

2. What are your personal obstacles to starting a new class or activity?

3. How important is social interaction in your life?

   VERY IMPORTANT     HERE AND THERE     NOT SO MUCH

4. Do you have any fears regarding any activities in your workplace? If so, how can you modify the activity to a lower degree of risk?

5. What is something you used to do and enjoy that you have not done in a long time?

6. Of these ten modules, which is a match for you to lead?

   Games    Outside    Hobbies    Food Prep

   Music    Spa    Exercise    In the Community

   Reading/Storytelling    Around the House

7. Do you have any suggestions regarding the schedule that could open up more opportunities for engagement?

8. Do you feel your job should not include doing engagement or that doing so is "impossible" with your other responsibilities?

9. List a few facts about your present day personhood:

   - 
   - 
   - 
   - 
   - 

10. Is an *engagement star* a healer?

# Section 3: Assistance

## "The Old Man and His Grandson"

from Grimm's Fairy Tales

*There was once a very old man, whose eyes had become dim, his ears dull of hearing, his knees trembled, and when he sat at the table he could hardly hold the spoon, and spilt the broth upon the tablecloth or let it run out of his mouth. His son and his son's wife were disgusted at this, so the old grandfather at last had to sit in the corner behind the stove, and they gave him his food in an earthenware bowl, and not even enough of it. And he used to look towards the table with his eyes full of tears. Once, too, his trembling hands could not hold the bowl, and it fell to the ground and broke. The young wife scolded him, but he said nothing and only sighed. Then they bought him a wooden bowl for a few half-pence, out of which he had to eat.*

*They were once sitting thus when the little grandson of four years old began to gather together some bits of wood upon the ground. 'What are you doing there?' asked the father. 'I am making a little wooden bowl,' answered the child, 'for father and mother to eat out of when I am big.'*

*The man and his wife looked at each other for a while, and presently began to cry. Then they took the old grandfather to the table, and henceforth always let him eat with them, and likewise said nothing if he did spill a little of anything.*

In this story of *transformation*, the husband and wife experience a drastic shift in perception. They have a realization that leads to compassion, from treating an elder as a nuisance to seeing him as a whole person again. The elder is accepted with his state of being exactly as it is. Persons with dementia have "a new normal that is different than it's been throughout their lives." (Lourdes 36)

The "new normal" is a level of ability at which a person needs increased assistance to be as healthy as possible. In person-centered care, the new normal becomes a "now normal" baseline of respected and valued levels of function. *Rementia* is promoted when current abilities are maximized. Providing assistance is good. Yet as the old saying goes: "Too much of a good thing is no longer a good thing."

## Assistant Defined

> **assist**—v. To help, support n. An act of giving aide, help. (*The American Heritage*, Fourth Edition)

A resident in a care community is a boss, and a caregiver is an assistant to the resident. The definition of assist does not include the words 'control,' 'decide for' or 'force.' A boss does not have assistants telling him what to do. An assistant who disregards the preferences of a boss is committing insubordination and is likely to be terminated. A boss has the final say.

A caregiver's job is to assist, not insist!

In this section, the discussion on assistance is not about how we safely transfer persons or provide incontinent care. Those skills are taught by licensed nurses, doctors, paramedics, clinicians, therapists, etc.… *REAL* explores how to respect personhood while providing services known as "activities of daily living" or "ADL's."

Section 2, *Engagement*, addressed appropriate activities to promote psychosocial well being. Person-centered assistance also promotes psychosocial well being. Rementia is possible when caregivers focus on the right amount of support to offer in all aspects of living. The objective is to blend person centered engagement and assistance with physical care needs (ADL's) into a synchronized relationship. All of the following terms represent **freedom to choose for one's self.**

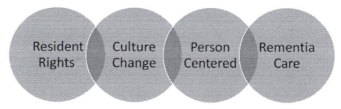

**Figure 3.1** All of the Above

All forms of assistance are opportunities to empower residents by promoting mental, emotional, and physical strength. Person-centered assistance is doing for a resident only what she is unable to do herself, encouraging her to participate, and giving her as much choice as possible in the process.

This section of the book may be challenging to get through. Readers are encouraged to approach the content with an open mind and a willingness to use what you can from the ideas presented. **I question standards and ask caregivers to take a soul-searching look at personal caregiving styles.** My belief in the power of caregivers as healers and in the transformation of care communities is why I have written this book.

## Doing, Doing, Doing

Throughout my years of experience, I have repeatedly seen the lack of time dedicated to address *psychosocial* needs. Whether in skilled nursing or assisted living centers, direct caregivers are expected to accomplish a tremendous list of tasks on each shift. We must find a new way to function and embrace a radical culture change to *transform* our communities.

Efficient personal care assistants, certified nurse aides, medication aides, licensed nurses, nurse managers, and housekeepers—staff who have the most contact with residents—are usually very detail oriented. They focus on tasks and go about their work in a structure designed to complete those tasks. **This is a good character trait.** Going about the daily routine with a 1, 2, 3, next, 1, 2, 3, next, mechanical approach *is not a bad way to function*, but a side effect is lack of attention to the population's general mood and level of satisfaction.

*Too much tasking negatively affects the overall environment.*

Residents are yearning for meaningful exchanges that do not happen when we are absorbed in busy-ness. Every instance of providing care is an opportunity for positive social interaction. During the doing, doing, doing, we can connect by asking personhood questions and explaining what we are doing and why we are doing it. Most importantly, we should show kindness and consideration in tone of voice, body language, and facial expressions.

> *It has become all too easy to ignore the suffering of a fellow human being, and see instead a merely biological problem, to be solved by some kind of technical intervention.* (Dr. Kitwood 44)

The source of the problem is how we have rated the importance of care duties. Productivity has been centered on physical and clinical needs while personhood has been overlooked. For many years, our quality of care standards have been based largely on *showers, grooming, and food consumption* without enough importance placed on the *number of laughs during lunch or the liveliness demonstrated during activities and residents' personal accomplishments.* The time has come to modify how we have "always" gone about our business in organized care settings.

In general, human beings are not quick to change, even when there is strong evidence change is needed. In long-term care communities, we have been out of balance, stuck in a framework of duties that does not allow enough space for meaningful activities. Nonetheless, we must find a way to meet the psychosocial needs of those we serve.

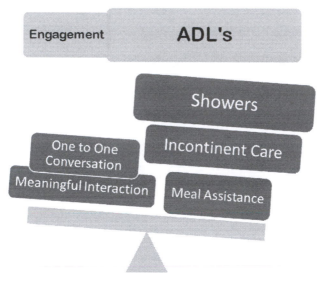

**Figure 3.2** No Time To Meet Psychosocial Needs?

All of those great engagement ideas in Section 2 will go nowhere if we stick to the conviction that engagement is secondary to meeting physical needs on a rigid schedule. Compromise on many levels is needed to do person-centered care with today's staffing models. We can do it.

Multiple reasons for not getting involved in engagement were considered in Section 2 of this guide. Time limitations were number one. Every member of the team must be truthful about all obstacles and be willing to experiment with alternate ways to go about the daily to do list. Corporate executives and owners are not likely to increase staffing ratios, yet regulations regarding personal preferences and psychosocial needs are more strictly enforced.

The president of the company where I was a program manager used the word "transformation" when describing his vision of engagement. He only approved raises if caregivers achieved high scores for engagement on evaluations. During interviews with potential caregivers, doing social activities with residents was emphasized, and the expectation was made clear. After I did training with the staff on engagement methods and developed the modular system, the personal care attendants found their own ways to do activities while still accomplishing the other "have to do's" of ADL assistance. Try the combinations below.

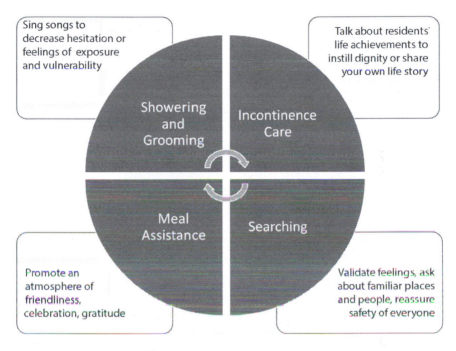

Sing songs to decrease hesitation or feelings of exposure and vulnerability

Talk about residents' life achievements to instill dignity or share your own life story

Showering and Grooming

Incontinence Care

Meal Assistance

Searching

Promote an atmosphere of friendliness, celebration, gratitude

Validate feelings, ask about familiar places and people, reassure safety of everyone

**Figure 3.3** During the Doing

## *Much To Do About Showers*

Perhaps a shower is not provided because a caregiver spent 20 minutes playing balloon volleyball with a group of residents who she spotted sitting in the hallway, still bodied and bored. She got an idea and blew up a balloon. For 20 minutes several people were alert, exercised with natural movements, and had many laughs hitting the balloon to each other. This scenario may not turn out well for the caregiver, who is perceived as goofing around. She may receive disciplinary action for not giving a shower. In "old-school" caregiving measures, playing with residents is not her job.

> *...speaking of activities, those that occur spontaneously are more meaningful to a resident than those for which they must wait for the scheduled time to come around. (Lourde 35)*

Am I suggesting we regularly skip showers to play balloon volleyball? No! However, the psychosocial needs of an unengaged group may have value equal to one resident's shower. I am suggesting a degree of flexibility in the daily schedule to open more windows for recreational activities and giving more credit to creative caregivers. Do we make a big issue about a missed shower, yet say nothing when a group of residents sit around for 30 minutes before dinner without any interaction?

Nancy Shier Anzelmo, of Alzheimer's Care Associates LLC, recommends showers to be scheduled only before breakfast and after dinner. Implementing this recommendation frees caregivers to do engagement while the whole community is awake. There are reasonable objections to this concept, such as:

> *How can I do all of my showers before breakfast and still have everyone up, dressed, and ready to go to the dining room in time?*

This is a legitimate concern, so we must consider alternative ways to structure meeting ADL needs and re-evaluate whether *what we have been viewing as necessary is actually necessary.* In addition, we should look at whether we cause more harm than good when providing ADL care, particularly regarding showers. Showers are a huge point of contention on various levels and across the board. Some residents are horrified by the process of having strangers take off their clothing to the point of complete nudity. The sensation of shower spray on sensitive skin may not be pleasant. Perhaps giving a shower to a person who resists, screams, and becomes combative will someday be considered a form of abuse to the resident and the staff member who is expected to complete a potentially catastrophic task.

I like what I read from a blogger on www.aging.com about bathing people with dementia:

> "*...many of the generation now in their 80s and 90s grew up with weekly baths— sometimes because they lived out on farms and water was too precious to waste. For others, that routine was just normal behavior...he or she is not going to die of some dreadful disease caused by "lack of bath" syndrome. For some elders, some fairly clean clothes and a weekly bath is what they consider enough. However, there are other issues to consider.*"

One of those considerations is incontinence. There are times when a shower is necessary to clean up, but not always. There are excellent peri-care products on the market to promote hygiene after toileting or an incontinent episode without a full on shower. Regarding partial bathing, nurse practitioner Jennifer Serafin gives this advice on the website www.caring.com:

"When taking care of your *parents bathing and cleansing needs*, I recommend the following: Daily cleansing should include the face, peri area (groin), under the breasts, under skin folds, and the arm pits. Peri-care or washing the privates may have to be done more frequently if your parent is incontinent and using diapers. Full body bathing can be *done less often*, as skin tends to become drier and more fragile as we age. Frequent bathing can cause dry skin, itchy skin, and irritation..."

During the 1990's, "sponge baths" were a BIG 'NO NO!' A Director of Nursing I worked with absolutely would not permit them, and inspectors from the Department of Health could write deficiencies for partial bathing. In recent years there has been a shift about this issue, though there may still be many "old-school" opinions that highly oppose.

A Director of Nursing once gave a talk to staff about *"Poverty of the Mind."* She explained that just as we have poverty in our living conditions, we can have poverty in our thoughts. Poverty is a state of not having enough, which usually results in a lower quality of living. Limited thinking, *poverty of the mind*, brings limited results. When we expand what is possible in our own minds we will create more of what is needed. *What we need is more time.* Solution-oriented thinkers unite! Direct caregivers and supervisors should brainstorm together for ideas. Management must support the rementia transformation with new policies and procedures.

Creative scheduling can be used to implement Schier-Anselmo's recommendation to assist with showers only before breakfast and after dinner. Staggered arrival and departure times for a few on the morning and night shifts creates an overlap that can make a big difference. Those who come in earlier would leave earlier with the hours of diminished staff at lower demand periods (before midnight and after lunch). In addition, nurse managers and administrators can ensure enough showers are scheduled for the night shift in the very early morning hours for early birds already awake. Here is what I came up with to create more open time:

| 7-3 | 8 CA's | Becomes | 6-2 | 2 CA's |
|-----|--------|---------|-----|--------|
| 3-11 | 8 CA's | | 7-3 | 6 CA's |
| 11-7 | 4 CA's | | 3-11 | 8 CA's |
| | | | 11-7 | 3 CA's |
| | | | 12-8 | 1 CA |

Now there are three additional CA's during the 7 a.m.-8 a.m. hour, which is commonly one of the busiest hours of the day. For one hour in the afternoon, staff is decreased by two and for one hour at night decreased by one. With staggered scheduling, showers and breakfast assistance are completed earlier with less strain, opening the day for person centered engagement!

Just one more note about showers. Not many people are accustomed to showering during the afternoon or early evening, particularly seniors who were occupied with farming or other responsibilities from sun up until darkness. We are not respecting years and years of personal routines by insisting on giving showers based on inflexible schedules. Shifting our mindsets to a personhood approach is the starting point of person-centered care. The shower business is one example of how to create time to meet other needs with a good game of balloon volleyball. ☺

## The Whole Picture—Assistance at the Highest Level

Assisting with activities of daily living is what we do all day long. Often we do them without engaging. Sometimes we assist with activities, yet we do so without connecting. *Engagement is connecting.*

When we believe relating to others and showing compassion makes a difference for everyone, person-centered care comes about naturally. To practice person-centered care, we partner with our residents, *transforming task action to interaction.* Residents are included in decisions. Assistance becomes engagement and engagement becomes assistance.

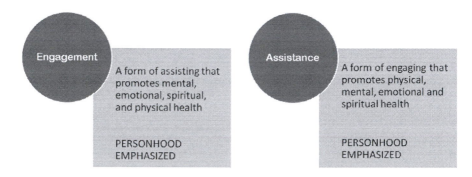

**Figure 3.4** Two of a Kind

The word transformation appears in the Nursing Home Quality Initiative of the Centers for Medicare and Medicaid Services:

"This initiative promotes the transformation of nursing facilities from institutional to person-centered care models." (CMS website)

Over ten years have passed since this initiative was published in 2002. *Are we providing person-centered care?* Each caregiver must answer this question for herself. We can look at an organization as a whole and make an overall judgment. We can give an opinion about our co-workers and what we see happening. Most effectively, though, is for each individual to do a thorough examination of her own approaches to resident care on a daily basis.

Rementia is transformation from a state of limited being to a state of whole existence. A major component of rementia is free will and respecting an individual's personhood and preferences. In person-centered care practices, we assist in restoring a resident's faith in his own being and in organized caregiving.

> *When a resident has an option about where he spends time, we promote freedom.*
> *When she is asked what she wants to wear, we promote freedom.*
> *When we give a choice about what he would prefer to eat, we promote freedom.*

Again, I refer to the brilliance of Dr. Kitwood, who named methods for providing care that nourish a person physically and emotionally. The following techniques exemplify master level caregiving skills. They are explained with more detail in *Dementia Reconsidered*. I have summarized the terms and added examples for demonstration:

> **Recognition**—Acknowledge a person, known by name, affirmed in his or her own uniqueness.
> *Greeting, careful listening, eye contact. I am the most guilty when it comes to walking by a person without saying hello. Dear, sweet Ivy was a great reminder for me with her "Slow down!" and "Well, hello to you, too!" as I sped through the corridor.*

> **Negotiation**—Consulting the person about preferences, desires, and needs rather than assuming a standard or common choice is correct. Negotiation takes into account anxieties and insecurities and gives power back to the individual receiving care.
> *Our goal should always be to help the resident get what they want or need (within reason), whether or not we fully understand why she wants it. Residents have rights! Resolve issues peacefully—never argue or confront.*

**Collaboration**—ADL's are not "done" to a person who is cast into a helpless role. Caregiving is a process wherein an individual takes initiative and uses her own abilities to a maximum extent.

*Our residents are whole beings. They do not need to be coddled or treated as if they are helpless. An example of collaboration is placing a fork in the hand of a person and allowing him to carry out the task of lifting to his mouth. Prompting with verbal cues is a form of collaboration. Collaboration is a method for completing conversations with results that have a resident feeling successful.*

**Play**—Spontaneous with no goal other than self-expression and fun. Many adults who have worked very hard and had stressful lives have not had much play time. A good care environment (rementing) promotes playful interaction.

*We are playful, real, and fostering the child within by having fun. Do those silly things we wouldn't do anywhere but in a Memory Care environment! What a great opportunity to be authentic without being judged!*

**Timalation**—Providing contact in a non-arousing yet stimulating way. Provide reassurance and pleasure in an honorable manner. Hugs, holding hands, gentle hand massages, and light kisses on the cheek. With severe cognitive impairment, this form of interaction is valuable.

*You have permission to love your residents. If you have reservations about touch, check with your supervisor and experienced caregivers about types of touch. Using the Spa module (Section 2) to do a gentle hand massage with lotion or a manicure are forms of timalation.*

**Celebration**—Any moment of life can be special and joyful. The division between a caregiver and the cared-for can completely vanish during celebration, as all are elevated to a higher mood.

*To lighten up in this environment, we need to celebrate every time we accomplish a goal together, have a breakthrough, or just share a special moment. When we have parties, we can really let go and feel the joy of living! Those we serve want us to feel happy at our work! They want to know we enjoy their company.*

**Relaxation**—Low level of intensity—slow pace. Some people with dementia are only able to relax when others are nearby or while having timalation (physical contact).

*Just being mellow is nice. Not everyone needs big doses of stimulation to be engaged. Knowing what brings each resident pleasure is the key. Relaxing engagement can be as simple as watching a sunset together.*

**Validation**—Acknowledging the person's emotions and feelings without arguing or trying to convince otherwise—giving a response on the feeling level. Understand the person's entire frame of reference (personal history, recent events, current mental age).

*Practice compassionate communication. When there is no immediate solution to a resident's seeking and/or anxiety, saying "I am sorry you are feeling so worried" or "This must be very tough for you." Authentic and caring statements acknowledge the feeling rather than the facts. Although we cannot fulfill some specific wishes, we can empathize with a feeling of loss, sadness or frustration. When we are genuine and use validation, our residents' personhood is supported. They will suffer less and experience more joy and peace.*

**Holding**—Provide a safe psychological space for intense emotional expression.

*If a resident appears to be emotionally upset, gently guide him out of a crowd to a quiet, comfortable place. Be sure to do this in a way that promotes dignity and respect. Let him express the feelings in a safe way, assuring him his feelings are important and that you will do whatever you can (within reason) to help. Know your own limitations and seek support from other staff or a supervisor if the situation seems to be worsening.*

**Facilitation**—To save time, we tend to do more than is necessary for a person—instead we must continue to see a person's strengths as greater than her disabilities and allow time for independence.

*Provide only those parts of the action that are missing. For example, encourage a resident to put on her own shirt. You only help with the buttons if she has trouble. Let her hold the hairbrush as you gently cup her hand and support the brushing motion. Place the washcloth in her hand to wash her face, and again, if necessary, cup hers with yours to support the process. Enable a person to get started and complete the task to the best of her ability.*

When caregivers practice the above methods, the entire mood of a care community will be lifted. Residents will be alive, alert, awake and enthusiastic. Staff members will feel successful. Rementia is a win-win prospect. To get there, we must eliminate some of the habits we have developed.

# Promoting the Decline in Well Being

Much of what we do now is person-centered care. However, much of what we do is not. We have learned from the mistakes of our past—like relying too heavily on medication and physical restraints to prevent "problem behavior." We have made great progress respecting resident rights and freedom of choice. For example, we learned that sherbet was not a wise substitute for ice cream after years of serving sherbet to people with diabetes who were asking for ice cream. Now we advise a person of the health risk and serve what they want.

Unfortunately, many providers are falling short in the **service** of recognizing and responding to feelings. When a caregiver fails to address emotional needs, a **disservice** has been committed. To ignore feelings because the cause is unknown or not real is to regard the person as not real.

> *Many cultures have shown a tendency to depersonalize those who have some form of serious disability (as though) those affected are not real persons.... Several factors come together to cause this dehumanization.* Dr. Kitwood p. 12

Dehumanization is a word that sounds very dramatic, almost gruesome. When I hear 'dehumanization,' I think of animals in an overcrowded shelter. There are bowls of food and water and litter boxes. Survival needs are met, but the animals are in cages. Unfortunately, that is how many view the long-term care scene—as a crude shelter for old people. Dr. Kitwood uses the word dehumanization to describe caregiving that is based on meeting only the physical needs of a person without regard for an individual's dignity.

While discussing living arrangement options, I said to an 86-year-old client of mine, "Assisted living is not a prison."

He responded, "No, but it's heading in that direction."

Yet since relocating to a memory-care development in an assisted living, he has been happily engaged and is grateful to be living in a simplified and accommodating arrangement.

We have come a long, long way in long-term care, and widespread practice of person-centered care will revamp our image into one where people will believe care communities are about freedom and healthy living.

Now and then people who have been in less than human environments, living in the street, or isolated at home alone and disabled, or with abusive/neglectful relatives, are placed in our care. They are grateful for three meals a day, a bed, electricity, heat and air conditioning, showers, people to talk to, and bingo with prizes. Organized care living is a huge improvement for those who have sat in their excrement for hours, hungry and afraid. One woman I recall arrived via Adult Protective Services. She was more than unclean—her hair was matted and stuck to her scalp. Thin, malnourished and dressed in rags, she had been living with family. In a few weeks she had gained weight and looked like a different person. She was a happy, pretty, remented woman. She was kind, sweet, and never complained at the nursing home.

A certain degree of rementia occurs just by meeting basic needs of food, shelter and medical attention when previously the needs were unmet. Yet we are striving to transform the whole picture and perception of who we are and what we are capable of achieving. I dream of the day when people will say, "Wow—long-term care communities do wonders!"

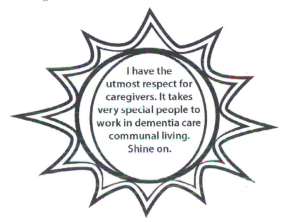

I have the utmost respect for caregivers. It takes very special people to work in dementia care communal living. Shine on.

Caregivers, please keep reading with an open mind and open heart. If you already excel in your work, this information will add to your gifts. Consider the possibilities.

Along with good habits, we all have bad habits. No one is perfect. Some of the habits we have developed in caregiving need to be broken. Are habits easy to change? Absolutely not. When we tend to the doing—the toileting, feeding, changing, transferring, showering—without taking time to really see the person we are helping, we are falling into poor work habits that developed out of busy routines, poor training or a lack of passion for this special occupation.

**When we cannot see upfront if a person is responding to us, we may have a tendency to forget about psychosocial needs.** We might think a smile makes no difference to the man who never smiles back. It does. We may believe a woman who seems only concerned with pacing the hallway is not impacted by our kind words. She is. We may feel we are wasting our time going the extra distance for someone who will not remember in five minutes. Not so. Every moment of connection we create is a healing moment.

## Old-School Caregiving

In person-centered care, we help residents get back some of what has been lost. Rementia. If we view dementia as the main feature of any person, we see limitation over capability.

When you have a cold and cannot get up from the couch, you are glad to have your loved ones take care of you. But you do not want to be treated as an out of touch person with no feelings. You would be offended if your loved ones gave no consideration to your preferences. You would feel shunned and ashamed if everyone stopped talking to you while you were sick. A person with an illness is still a complete person.

**As a society, we tend to treat persons with dementia as less than a whole human being:**

> *Caregivers who assume Mrs. Smith cannot brush her own teeth and hurriedly brush them for her to save time have given up on her abilities.*
> *Caregivers who do not consult with Mrs. Rodriguez about where she is being taken are leaving her out of her own life.*
> *Caregivers who talk over Mr. Jones while spooning soup into his mouth are announcing that Alzheimer's has won, and Mr. Jones has lost.*

In the above examples, caregivers are 'doing' without considering the person's deeper needs—the unseen, psychosocial need to be a part of what is happening around her and to her. The more we diminish a person's abilities by overlooking her capabilities, the more we **contribute to the decline of a person with dementia.** Dr. Kitwood describes these actions as a "social model of disability" (Dr. Kitwood p. 46) wherein persons are denied any say in what happens to them, unable to or discouraged from showing any power over a situation. Even more powerful is his description of the 'old culture of care' as one of "malignant social psychology." (Dr. Kitwood 46)

When the first long-term care centers were opened, there was limited information available to caregivers about the residents' conditions. The level of fear must have been tremendous. Fear is a powerful emotion that spreads like a virus of the spirit. We often fear what we do not understand and act out of the instinct to protect ourselves and others. The first hospitals designed to treat persons with thought disorders had policies and procedures based on A LOT OF FEAR. Though we are now better educated to make decisions, the culture of care based on fear still dominates. Overcoming history and the cruel treatment of those with mental health conditions has been underway in the United States for several decades. Yet the failure to regard those with dementia as whole persons is a social model of disability and malignant social psychology that prevails.

> *The word malignant signifies something very harmful, symptomatic of a care environment that is deeply damaging to personhood, possibly even undermining physical well-being....The term malignant does not, however, imply evil intent on the part of caregivers; most of their work is done with kindness and good intent. The malignancy is part of our cultural inheritance. (Dr. Kitwood 46)*

Dr. Kitwood is saying caregivers are good-hearted people who mean well and do not want to cause harm or injury. The definitions of abuse and neglect in the eyes of a long-term care surveyor include the words "intention to cause harm." Intention means committing an action known to cause damage with presence of mind while doing so. Physical abuse and neglect are usually not hard to identify. But whether or not a resident has been emotionally neglected or psychologically hurt by a caregiver can be very difficult to determine.

Unknowingly, without intention, or as a means to complete tasks quickly, we may be conducting ourselves in a manner that *does not serve our residents well. We believe ourselves to be efficient, completely unaware that the methods we use add to the chaos, confusion or disability.* People did not know smoking was bad for our health until the results of smoking became apparent, often too late to recover. With malcaregiving, actions may not appear harmful. Caregivers may be providing malignant care without realizing the negative side effects. The damage occurs on the inside of the resident, just as it does with someone who smokes.

## Malcaregiving Habits

Even the best caregivers may be unaware of poor habits that cause further damage to a person whose self worth has been compromised by a disease process. Dr. Kitwood wrote of 17 techniques that contribute to the decline of a person with dementia. Below are definitions with examples of seven actions I have observed most frequently. *There is no blame in this process, only opportunities to learn.*

> **Disempowerment**—failing to encourage a person to use the abilities they do have; failing to help them to complete actions they have initiated. (Dr. Kitwood 46)

*To ignore that a person is able to pull up his own pants and to do it for him to save time is to treat him as less than whole. We are undermining personhood when we do not give him the chance to exercise his ability. Let him do as much as he can independently and support by finishing the task, such as fastening the button.*

**Infantilization**—treating a person very patronizingly as an insensitive parent might treat a very young child. (Dr. Kitwood 46)
*Tone of voice and word choice makes the difference between healthy guidance and malcaregiving. Scolding, warning, or "talking down" to a resident is demeaning and a form of emotional abuse. Always communicate concerns with respect.*

> *Stop that or you will get hurt!*

> *I am afraid you may get hurt, please stop.*

**Outpacing**—providing information, presenting choices, etc. at a rate too fast for a person to understand; putting them under pressure to do things more rapidly than they can bear. (Dr. Kitwood 47)
*Ask simple questions with one option as an answer, such as "Would you like orange juice?" rather than "Do you want milk or water or orange juice?" Pushing someone in a wheelchair faster than that person would be walking is a form of physical outpacing, as is rushing someone to get ready or to move from one location to another too quickly.*

**Invalidation**—failing to acknowledge the subjective reality of a person's experience, and especially what they are feeling. (Dr. Kitwood 47)
*Validation is to acknowledge feelings instead of arguing about facts. Never tell a person with dementia he should not feel how he feels or try to talk a person out of what he believes. Find a connection between the situation at hand and the feelings being expressed.*

> *Don't cry. That's not your wife leaving. Your wife died many years ago.*

> *Does her long, dark hair remind you of your wife's hair? You must miss her.*

**Objectification**—treating a person as if they were a lump of dead matter; to be pushed, lifted, filled, pumped or drained, without proper reference to the fact that they are sentient beings. (Dr. Kitwood 47)
*A disturbing example of objectification is "feeding" residents in a hurried and impersonal manner. Persons who require assistance are still able to enjoy the act of eating. Residents who can eat independently with cues are*

*to be verbally encouraged and prompted, as earlier described in the term "facilitation." The process may be slow and messy. Slow down, make eye contact, and talk to the person you are assisting.*

**Ignoring**—carrying on (in conversation or action) in the presence of a person as if they were not there. (Dr. Kitwood 47)
*Discussing what is to be done without communicating to the person to whom the action is being done is beyond inconsiderate. Talking over residents without including them in conversations is neglecting the need for belonging. The mark we leave may not be a visible, but overlooking the presence of a person is like a slap in the face. Caregiving is about the feelings behind the face, not just washing the face!*

**Imposition**—forcing a person to do something, overriding desire or denying the possibility of choice on their part. (Dr. Kitwood 47)
*Residents wheeled down the hall not in favor of the trip or not knowing where they are going is a form of imposition. Use a pleasant tone of voice to explain what is happening and why it is necessary. Unless a resident is in immediate or obvious danger, one should never be pushed, pulled, argued with or unfairly convinced to do anything.*

Come on Mr. Jones, let's go to the recreation room!

Mr. Jones, would you like to go to the recreation room? I think you will like the people there.

**Disruption**—intruding suddenly or disturbingly upon a person's action or reflection, crudely breaking their frame of reference. (Dr. Kitwood 47)
*Control the impulse to rush a person who is speaking. Allow time to communicate. If a resident is having a conversation with another person, wait until a pause to speak about what needs to be accomplished. Ask for permission to interrupt. In care communities, common courtesy should be the practice.*

In Section 4 of this guide, I have recorded numerous expressions of love personally witnessed from caregivers to residents. There is so much awesome caregiving happening. But how often do you hear "she's a feeder" right in front of the woman who needs assistance eating or "put him there" about the man in a wheelchair? Those expressions are used to increase effectiveness in delivering services, but they are insensitive to the residents. Strong words such as "malcaregiving" and "dehumanization" should not be used lightly.

However, when poor care practices are the accepted norm, residents are 'dehumanized':

> *In this kind of way we move towards a 'neurology of personhood.' All events in human interaction—great and small—have their counterpart at a neurological level… A malignant social psychology may actually be damaging to nerve tissue….Maintaining personhood is both a psychological and a neurological task. (Dr. Kitwood 19)*

When we perform services—dressing, transferring, and showering—without seeing the person we are helping as fully present, we are causing psychological damage that contributes to a downward direction of dementia. Acknowledging personhood during ADL's promotes rementia. Taking the extra measures involved in person-centered techniques is time well spent.

## Mealtime Opportunities

Ensuring a person with dementia is in the right place at the right time and receiving the right level of assistance to get a full belly is the most important responsibility we have as caregivers. But we also need to consider: How are we engaging during the meal? Are we promoting a resident centered environment while the meal is consumed? What social needs are being met while eating? You may be asking:

> *Just what does this woman want us to do? Sing and dance while we pass trays?*

Well, if you can carry a tune, and there is no music in the dining room….

SHOUT OUT TO HARDWORKING CAREGIVERS READING THIS: You have a tough role and are admired for what you do. Just a reminder that texting during mealtimes is not acceptable. Neither is talking to your fellow CNA about what you did last night. Make conversation with the person you are assisting. That's person-centered care and it doesn't take any more time or energy. **Be present to your residents.**

As a caregiver, I am guilty at times of engaging with co-workers over residents. My psychosocial needs include knowing my co-workers. Let's offer our care partners gentle reminders when we are spending too many minutes with attention away from the ladies and gentlemen who are our customers. Habits are hard to break. Transformation will occur when enough of us are willing to take a close look and make changes that promote *engagement*.

Many years have passed since the introduction of resident rights, mandatory training, and company campaigns on culture change. Yet I continue to observe staff treating residents as objects during mealtimes almost everywhere I work, visit, do training or volunteer. On my last assignment, it took many reminders for the staff to routinely ask "soup or salad?"—offering a choice instead of assuming that it did not matter to the resident. By holding a soup in one hand and a salad in the other, the resident can nod or reach if unable to speak.

I am an advocate of staff members joining the residents for meals at a "family table," which is what I renamed the "feeder table"—where residents who benefit from prompting and aid are seated. Spending just 15 minutes at the "family table," promotes visual cueing and the social aspect of having a guest adds incentive to eat. Persons who barely touch their food will eat more when they see others enjoying the food. So the caregiver eats, but this time does not count as her break.

Although music during mealtimes creates a nice atmosphere, the volume and selection should compliment the environment. Television should only be on if a resident has made the request and the selection is pleasant for everyone to watch. Conversation between table mates is the best form of engagement and more likely with lower noise levels. Avoid yelling about meals and mistakes. Consider the dining room to be a nice restaurant. Residents are paying customers.

**Rementia challenge to management:**

> *Be of service for 15 minutes during any meal three days a week.*
> *Help serve or clear tables or join in at the family table.*
> *Engage before or during the meal.*
> *Is it fair to expect direct caregivers to squeeze more time out of their busy schedules to engage if administration is not willing to do the same?*

Remember your *REAL* purpose.

## Searching for the Familiar

Searching is commonly referred to as "sun downing," "exit-seeking," and "wandering." I call this compulsion "searching" because the person attempting to leave or constantly pacing is likely to be looking for someone or something familiar and may have time travelled into the past. Such is the case in the story of Ivy in Section 1. Searching can be due to a physical condition, such as hunger or a bathroom need. Identifying cause and soothing a person obsessed with searching is one of the most time consuming aspects of providing dementia care.

A common approach is to "distract" or "re-direct" the searcher with simple solutions such as offering a drink of water or food. Re-direction as such can work in some instances if the problem is actually hunger or thirst. From personal experience, distracting and re-directing are not usually effective when a person is bent on finding that familiar person, place or thing. The person searching may stay in a piano performance for a few minutes, and then she is off again. Handling a searching spell may require concentrated one-to-one attention while applying validation techniques. Unfortunately, all too often the searching behavior is ignored or downplayed, and the resident is abandoned in a state of anxiety and fear.

> *Residents are full human beings who have experienced a radical, frightening shift in perception, and their 'difficult behaviors' are their attempt to gain their footing, achieve control, cope with stressors, problem-solve, and communicate unmet needs. (Lourde 24)*

What is the emotion underneath the searching? Ask the resident to talk about her life to determine what age she is remembering. If she is attempting to leave, is there a way to demonstrate the danger of exiting? For example, look out the window together to see if there is anything familiar outside. Show her photos of her family and reassure her they are safe right now. About that missing purse, call the front desk as she listens, and assure her it will be turned in when found.

What is commonly called "sun downing" is a phenomenon occurring in late afternoon. That is the time of day when kids get out of school, moms change focus, people get off work—the mood of the day is changing as we head into an evening at home. Perhaps the increase in exit seeking is due to a shift in responsibilities from one location to another. Maybe sensing that darkness will come soon plays a part in the instinct to be in a safe, familiar place. How we respond to the searching before, during, and after sundown is more important than the cause.

Has it ever happened that early in the day a woman in a care community was searching and no one stopped to explore her concerns by using validation methods? Twenty minutes might have done the trick. Has it ever happened that after a few hours of unsuccessful searching, she began screaming that she was going to "get out of here," yet still no one found time to connect with her? Twenty minutes might have resolved her angst. Did staff continue to brush it off saying "she does that a lot" when twenty minutes could turn her around? Continuing, has it ever happened that this woman was sent out on a 911 emergency because she became "a harm to herself and others," combative when staff stopped her forceful exit through the alarmed door?

It takes more than twenty minutes to deal with a 911 incident. How much staff time was spent describing the situation to the operator, the police, fire, and ambulance responders, notifying the director, doing paperwork, copying records, and calling the family? Furthermore, the crisis was traumatizing for the woman, compounding her feeling that she has no control over anything in her life as she is strapped down to a gurney. In her reality, this is happening because she could not find her kids or car or purse. She feels persecuted. It does not make sense to her, and it is indeed senseless.

True stories like this may worsen a person's state of dementia and could be the result of malcaregiving. Enough said about errors of our over-tasking, get-it-done, hurried ways. Malcaregiving is heavy stuff that can be tough to digest. Our direction is toward rementia.

Being a good caregiving assistant is exhaustingly hard work. Providing person-centered care is not about making the job harder. It is about lifting the job higher.

As a result of the 1987 Omnibus Reconciliation Act (OBRA '87) regulatory requirements were passed regarding psychosocial, functional, behavioral, and quality of life issues for long-term care residents. Outcomes from meeting physical needs, such as a shower, are objective quality indicators. Judging how well psychological needs are met is subjective and not as easy to measure. However, a reduction in reported incidences resulting in injury or discharges due to "harmful behavior" can be tracked over a period of time.

The old saying "An ounce of prevention is worth a pound of cure" applies here, and the prevention strategy is person-centered care assistance. The cure is an outcome: rementia. **We do not have to wait for scientific evidence to move ahead with rementia theory.** The healing can start now with intention to transform. Together we can discover new ways to create well being through appropriate forms of assistance.

# TILT Keys on Assistance

1. What ideas do you have about scheduling that could open up time for more engagement while supporting physical ADL's?

2, What is your understanding of the concept "malcaregiving?"

3, How would you feel if every time a resident was ignored the overhead speaker made a loud buzzing sound? Would it be noisy in your care community?

4, Rank the actions according to how often you observe them in your care community, with 1 being the most and 7 the least.

| | |
|---|---|
| DISRUPTION | _____ |
| OUTPACING | _____ |
| IGNORING | _____ |
| INVALIDATING | _____ |
| DISEMPOWERMENT | _____ |
| INFANTILIZATION | _____ |
| OBJECTIFICATION | _____ |

5. Would poor work habits decrease if staff could see neuron function decreasing in a resident's brain immediately following an act of malcaregiving?

6. Give an example of how to say "Don't be sad that your daughter left" without invalidating the emotion of sadness:

7. Without free will, what would your life be like?

8. Are you willing to slow down and examine your own caregiving actions?

9. Will you take a stand to support transformation in your workplace by demonstrating and sharing person-centered care techniques?

10. What is the most rewarding aspect of your job as a caregiver?

# Section 4: Love

## And the Greatest of These Is Love

"I'M GOING HOME TODAY!"

Belle spoke these words over and over after moving into the assisted living memory care community. She was not happy. As her distress increased, so did the mild panic attacks for which she was prescribed an anti-anxiety medication. Her family was considering moving her to another care community.

"What do you miss about home, Belle?"

"I miss my stuff. They're living in my house, and they're not taking care of my stuff."

"Can you show me some stuff in your room?"

Belle and I would go to her room and look at the pictures, her furniture, the paintings, and knick knacks. We would talk about the history of her belongings. Sometimes our talk would help, other times she would not let go of going home.

One day, when she repeatedly talked about leaving I said, "Belle, you just can't go home today. I'm sorry. Dr. Denise wants you to stay here for a while longer."

"Okay," she sighed. "What about tomorrow?"

"I don't know what will happen tomorrow."

"Then I am going home tomorrow!" At least that was progress.

Keeping Belle occupied was a good challenge—like many people with moderate AD, she had boundless energy and liked to stay busy. For Christmas I gave her a green and white polka dotted broom, and when she was feeling restless, I would ask her to sweep. She would do a thorough job. From the housekeeping module, she used soapy rags to wipe down the dining room chairs. "We need more hot water!" she would exclaim. Much of her personhood was based on being a dedicated mother and good housewife.

Belle could still bathe and dress herself and only needed reminders to brush her hair or change clothes. She was continent and ate very well on her own. **Her psychosocial needs were greater than her physical needs**. She had a very large and fun loving Italian family. Giving and receiving affection remained a huge part of her personhood.

One day during a musical performance, the singer was performing *I Can't Help Falling In Love With You* (Weiss, Creatore, Peretti). I waltzed over to Belle, looked her straight in the eyes and sang to her. To this she replied:

"Okay, maybe I will stay. But I have to go get my stuff." My heart melted. She stopped talking about going home, and as rementia grew stronger, she stopped talking about getting her stuff too. She even developed a romance with a male resident. Several months later, Belle died, having spent her last days happy and content in a care community.

This poem was written for Belle:

*You won my heart, and then gave me yours*
*I missed you on my days off, and I miss you now*
*You went to join Frankie, dancing in the starry streets*

## Incredible Caregivers

Many are the expressions of love I have witnessed from caregiver to care receiver. Those who continue to serve in this field are undoubtedly the most exemplary persons in the world. Through the years I have seen caregivers do the following and so much more:

*Using their own lunch breaks to go purchase food, with their own money, for residents who mentioned how much they missed a burger and fries, tacos, or fried chicken.*

*Using their personal time and money, buying Christmas presents and ordinary items such as a nightgown or socks for someone who has no family.*

*Using their own money for vending machine treats for residents.*

*Bringing movies from home or renting a requested favorite for residents to watch.*

*Coming in on her day off to bring Birthday flowers.*

*Visiting residents in the hospital off the clock.*

*Attending funeral services and memorials off the clock.*

*Hugging, blowing kisses, and declaring "You're my special lady!" or "I love you!"*

*Gently rubbing a resident's feet in the morning to ease her into waking up.*

Out of respect for direct caregivers I formed a nonprofit organization, FutureCare Now, Inc., with the mission statement to "Recruit, retain and recognize" staff in long-term care settings. FutureCare Now held an annual "Long-term Care Awareness Fair." The public was invited to learn about care companies, receive free health screenings, and witness a recognition ceremony. Nominees from nursing facilities throughout San Antonio were awarded inscribed plaques, gift cards, and event T-shirts for their labors of love.

> *Love wasn't put in your heart to stay.  Love isn't love until you give it away.*
> Anonymous

Caregivers are exceptional people. On any given shift, a caregiver may walk into the room of a woman with whom she has spent many days and find the woman still, eyes open, last words spoken. The caregiver remains calm, perhaps says a little prayer, feels a sense of loss and wonder—then notifies a supervisor and continues on assisting others without missing a beat.

## The Healing Power of Love

Love is the greatest power on earth. Love transforms care communities into healthy and loving environments. We need more nursing homes and assisted living residences to be regarded as healthy and loving models of care. In the progression of long-term care models, we are seeing a significant shift in quality of care and *meeting social needs along with providing clinical services.* We are beginning to be viewed in a brighter light.

*Love*—n. Strong affection; warm attachment; unselfish, loyal and benevolent concern for others  (Merriam Webster Dictionary)

The proceeding three sections of this guide have been about how to practice person-centered care and how to promote rementia. The growing emphasis on psychosocial needs has opened space for caregivers to express who we are as unique individuals and to explore what we have in common with those we serve—the capacity to give and receive love.

The first section of this book "Rementia," is an introduction to the concept of restoring personhood. The second section "Engagement," is about stimulating the mind and body with appropriate levels of activity. The third section "Assistance," focuses on how to meet physical needs of the body with respect for a person as a whole being. The final section is "Love," a spiritual aspect of caregiving. When we bring engagement, appropriate level of assistance, and love together, we have a complete care model for the mind, body, and spirit.

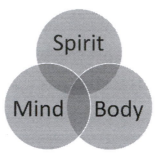

**Figure 4.1** The Rementia Recipe

Meeting the mental, physical, and spiritual needs of those we serve are equally important. They require different kinds of strength from caregivers. I know of no other occupation with such complexity. Caregivers who accomplish complete care deserve a standing ovation at the end of each shift.

## Coming from Love When We Get Busy

For transformation to occur in 24-hour care settings, healing through love must occur on a large-scale profound level. We can practice acts of love not just toward our residents. That means adoring our co-workers—every single one. When love permeates all we do, good mental, physical, and spiritual health will flourish.

> *Like many others, I discovered that intense involvement with people who have dementia and their carers makes heavy emotional demands. There is a great deal of anxiety and distress, and at times it feels as if one might sink into a vast morass of unmet need. (Dr. Kitwood 5)*

Showing affection enhances person-centered care and promotes well being. Too often the feeling of love gets lost when the demands of the job are heavy, which is most of the time. Feeling overburdened, caregivers often become overly focused on the next task at hand and providing services with affection is compromised. **Under stress, connecting with residents can be buried among all there is to do.**

A caregiver who feels rushed to complete a shower in time to start the meal service can benefit by slowing down for a moment, taking a few deep breaths and affirming: ***"I express love through my thoughts, actions and words."***

## Assisting with Emotional State

Human beings are human beings at all ages and during all stages of life. Throughout our years, we seek validation of our physical and emotional needs. We have feelings from the moment we are delivered from the womb until the moment we receive our last breath. Until then, our emotional needs lay waiting to be fulfilled. Even the seemingly distant spirit may appreciate simple pleasures, like that of a gentle touch and a reassuring voice. From the beginning of life, we seek to love and be loved, for this is the essence and the truth of who we are here to be.

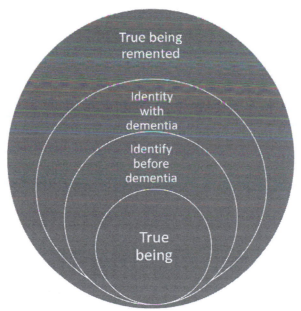

**Figure 4.2** Return to True Being

When a person is suffering, good caregivers have a natural instinct to respond with love. The following techniques are examples of master caregiving. From Dr. Kitwood's masterpiece, *Dementia Reconsidered,* the following are summaries and examples of five concepts: **comfort, attachment, inclusion, occupation, and identity**.

> **Provide Comfort**—Show tenderness, closeness. Sooth the pain and sorrow. Reduce anxiety. "To comfort a person is to provide a kind of warmth and strength which might enable them to remain in one piece when they are in danger of falling apart." (Dr. Kitwood 81)
> *Perhaps the man being assisted to the table could use an extended moment of eye contact to break a feeling of loneliness.*

> **Show Attachment**—Form bonds, safety nets. "Without the reassurance that attachments provide it is difficult for any person, of whatever age, to function well." (Dr. Kitwood 82)
> *Let your residents know their well-being is important to you. Express concern.*

> **Make Everyone Feel Included**—Our species is social and designed for face-to-face communication. "The need for inclusion comes…in so called attention-seeking behavior…" (Dr. Kitwood 83) Individuals need to have a distinct place in the shared life of our population.
> *Could it be the new resident is feeling uneasy and needs re-introduction to tablemates? Is self-introduction a part of group activities?*

> **Create Occupation**—To be occupied is the opposite of feeling bored or hopeless. Real engagement is about occupation whether working on a project or playing. "If people are deprived of occupation their abilities began to atrophy, and self-esteem drains away. The need for occupation is still present in dementia…it takes a great deal of skill and imagination to meet the need without imposing false solutions." (Dr. Kitwood 83)
> *Ask residents to help with simple tasks. Remember, it is not important for the resident to do the task accurately or completely. Always say "Thank you for your help!"*

> **Recognize Identity**—"To have an identity is to know who one is…" (Dr. Kitwood 83) Regardless of how much a person can recall about his personhood, we continue to honor him as whole, with a full life, past and present.
> *When serving that drink of water, use the resident's name: "Here you go, Mr. Williams."*

## What Keeps Us from Total Love?

"Old-school" teaching and training put limits on how intimate we could be with residents. Maybe this was to avoid misinterpretation of our intentions. Perhaps it was because showing love is thought to take too much time and energy and may detract from clinical responsibilities. Many times I have heard criticism amongst peers for being emotionally close to residents.

> *They have a fear factor. The state says you cannot touch them in an inappropriate way, and you get it through your nurses' training where you have to create a space between you and your patients.—Jayne Clairmont, owner and operator of English Rose Suites (Lourde 28)*

There are nurses who were taught to put up emotional barriers to prevent personal attachment to patients. Keeping a distance between their "selves" and the patients' "selves" was to maintain a "professional" relationship. There may be certain nurse to patient relationships where this tactic is necessary. However, while serving persons with Alzheimer's disease and all forms of dementia, a bond of love supports well being on both sides of the caring.

Another reason for the detached style of caregiving may be "old-school" mentality wherein caregivers are viewed as authority figures. Such theory stems from the belief that if one is too kind or friendly, the resident may not be cooperative. This attitude may be an excuse for controlling an individual and has no place in person-centered care.

We must search deep within to uncover psychological reasons for withholding our feelings of love. Perhaps there is a fear that if we give our hearts fully we will be hurt by our residents' actions, illnesses, or imminent deaths. The caregiver dance is a delicate balance of letting people in and letting go.

In the book "The English Patient," by Michael Ondaatje, the main character, Hana, is a young nurse during World War II. The author describes Hana's thoughts:

"Throughout the war, with all of her worst patients, she survived by keeping a coldness hidden in her role as nurse." Hana says, "I will survive this. I won't fall apart at this." (Ondaatje p.48) At another point in the story, she has the thought "Who the hell were we to be given this responsibility, expected to be wise as old priests, to know how to lead people towards something no one wanted and somehow make them feel comfortable." (Ondaatje p. 84)

Though Hana is a fictional character, I relate to her. When I worked for the Alzheimer's Association, we used the phrase "The War on Alzheimer's." I have felt tremendous grief over the decline and loss of a resident and agree that we must remain emotionally strong lest we abandon the cause altogether. However, to continuously put up a barrier to preserve one's own self-image is not in the best interests of rementia. The progression of AD can be very painful to witness, yet being connected to the affected person is critical for a peaceful resolution in the end. We embrace the process with love even when we are afraid.

## Love Is Letting Go of Fear

To walk through fear, we trust in the life process, holding each other and every aspect of the work environment in the light. Despite the past or our pre-set conceptions, we have faith that all will work out as meant to be. Once we develop trust, we have greater access to the love within our hearts and the hearts of those we serve.

*Your part is not to wonder how love works, but just to dare to begin releasing it from within yourself.*
(Ponder 18)

People with Alzheimer's often have unwarranted suspicions and delusional beliefs. Frequently caregivers are unfairly accused and blamed for circumstances difficult to explain to someone with dementia. We may feel betrayed by someone we care about, and continuing to come from love can be difficult. Instead we become defensive and perhaps angry. Sometimes we are physically attacked and verbally assaulted. Naturally, we feel hurt and disrespected.

At these times, we must remember that the person for whom we are caring has a thought disorder. As hard as it can be, we must look beyond the illness and continue to practice the art of compassion. We must recognize that we are dealing with profound confusion.

Through the moments of misunderstanding, when both giver and receiver are frustrated, we can recall the *transformative* quality of love.

> *Stop thinking of dementia patients as people with diseases to be treated, and start thinking of them as people with a terrifying, shifted reality who still have lots left to give if their trust can just be earned. (Lourde 22)*

When I began the garden engagement with Mr. Williams (Section 1), he believed himself to be back in basic training with the Air Force. He would say, "This is my room until I get transferred to another unit," or "I'm not sure how long I am going to be in this program, but I'll help you as long as I can." I would accept his perception and ask him to help just for today.

During the course of writing this book, I had an interesting dream. I was driving along and came to a toll booth where I had to show proof of my legal age. I did not have an I.D. with me. The woman in the booth asked my age, and I responded, "Well, I am not sure, but I think I am old enough." I remember how strange it felt *not to be able* to recall my age. In a mirror behind the woman's desk, I saw my reflection as younger than I am now. I said to the woman, "What do you think? I must be getting close to 30." She agreed and allowed me to pass.

In the morning, I recalled the dream—the feeling of uncertainty, the confusion of not knowing my own age. CLEARLY, WRITING THIS BOOK WAS GETTING TO ME. The dream gave me a sense of how strange memory loss must feel, particularly losing facts about one's own personhood.

The "time travelling" aspect of Alzheimer's disease is fascinating. As a nightly dreamer, I can sympathize with those who are confused about *where they are, how they got there, and why they are there*. My dreams are full of scenes where I am looking for my children, late to school or work, or forgetting important responsibilities. Frequently I dream of being lost on a highway somewhere, desperately trying to figure out how to get home.

My anxiety dreams sound like scenarios we often hear from residents. Gratefully, I wake up from my dreams. How can we help our residents, in a gentle, non-abrasive manner, have a shift from the panic of a living nightmare to feeling safe and settled? Love is the answer. To nurture others, our sense of love must be infallible. Love includes honoring our own personhood.

## Self-Care—Give Yourself Love

Being employed as a healer requires tremendous energy and stamina. There should be a basic training program to maximize physical strength and mental conditioning before caregivers work the floor. Most people have no idea just how hard this job is going to be when they enter the long-term care arena. Unprepared for the level of stress, many people do not make it for long.

> *Interestingly, two reports from nursing homes found that staff experienced more stress when caring for patients with dementia. (Jennings 2)*

Those who continue on for months and years seem to have a higher tolerance for stress. However, working under demanding conditions for a prolonged period can have negative effects on even the best of caregivers. All too often, lifestyle choices do not support ongoing exposure to the pressure in caregiving, especially providing for those with forms of dementia. How can we be loving, patient, and kind if we feel worn out by stress?

> *They have a difficult job, often a thankless one. Working day after day with residents who cannot carry on a conversation, say thank you, or remember their caregivers is not easy. Resident deaths are a fact of life, yet there is often little or no time to grieve…. Some family members direct the frustration and anger evoked by the disease toward the nurses and direct-care staff. So, just as the residents need special care, so too, do the staff. (Simard 54)*

The term "burnout," describes a condition in which a person is no longer performing at full capacity due to the strain of meeting job expectations. Unfortunately, many caregivers continue working with low level burn out. In this condition, a caregiver has either consciously or unconsciously given up on doing his best. Perhaps due to physical pain or mental exhaustion, he is no longer able to do all that is required. Either way, the minimal amount of work is completed on each shift—enough to stay in good standing and hold the position. He feels defeated by the terms of continued employment, yet needs the job for income. In this state of indifference the caregiver has become desensitized to the deeper needs of the residents. Although he may genuinely love the residents, showing affection has become difficult due to apathy.

Many workplace factors that lead to stress and burnout are not in the caregiver's control. However, individuals can make healthy lifestyle choices to promote stress management and well being. Increased stress can lead to unhealthy behaviors such as smoking, comfort eating, poor diet choices, inactivity and drinking alcohol or taking illicit drugs. Heavy reliance on junk food and substances can lead to long-term, serious health problems. Try these strategies for managing your work-related stress:

- **Be aware of your stress level.** What are the signs your stress level is increasing? Do you lose patience with your family or coworkers or residents when you feel overwhelmed by work pressures? Do you have a hard time concentrating or making decisions? Do you have chronic headaches, muscle tension or a lack of energy? Learn your own stress signals and how you deal with them to avoid falling into unhealthy patterns of behavior.

- **Use your cell phone or a notepad to keep a "To-Do" list.** Are you anxious about all the tasks you need to complete on your shift and afraid you will forget something important? Use those electronic devices as tools for organization and time management. Set alarms to remind you that a resident is waiting in the bathroom or that your break time is coming up. If your company has a policy about carrying cell phones on the clock, be a part of the solution by showing managers what functions can help you improve job performance. Be sure the ring tones selected are not offensive or loud enough to cause a disturbance.

- **Take stretching and breathing breaks.** Take a minute throughout the day to stretch, breathe deeply and shake off the accumulating tension between tasks, before moving on to the next. Only sacrifice break times for life or death emergencies. If you cannot find someone to cover for you, inform your supervisor. If break times are regularly missed by many employees, and you have reported following the chain of command without resolution, write notes to the administrator or executive director until the system is fixed.

- **Find healthy ways to manage stress.** Make an effort to replace unhealthy foods, smoking, or drinking alcohol with healthy behaviors, like eating fresh fruits, exercising, and meditation or prayer. Bad habits develop over time and can be difficult to change, so pick one at a time and focus on changing that one. Some behaviors may require the help of a support group, physician or psychologist. Meeting schedules can be found at www.oa.org. for overeaters anonymous, www.na.org. for narcotic abuse, and www.aa.org. for alcohol abuse. These free programs are open to anyone who is interested in a better way of living and have for decades proven that people can beat their unhealthy addictions. Caregivers can attend support groups to share and learn from other caregivers. See www.alz.org.

- **Develop a caring lifestyle.** Eat right, get enough sleep, drink plenty of water and do stretching to unwind those muscles that work so hard on the job. Even after the hardest day, lying on the floor to do gentle movements extending your spine and limbs should feel good. Practice deep breathing exercises. No matter how hectic life gets, make time to let go and relax.

- **Take the vacation time you have earned.** Money is tight, so many caregivers opt to cash in their paid time off rather than take much needed days away from the job. Consider taking at least half of your accumulated hours off to spend time with family, take a short trip, even for the day, or stay home and watch favorite movies to catch up on rest.

Caregivers often fail to meet their own personal needs. The nurse aide says to a resident's wife, "You'd better go home and rest or you might not make it here tomorrow." Then the nurse aide agrees to work a double, wears herself thin, picks up a burger and fries on the way home and collapses on the couch. Good nurse aide, take your own advice. Be your own healer first and foremost. Then your love and good works can flow.

## Co-workers Cooperating

One meaning of the prefix "co" is "together." Working together we are joined as partners toward a mutual goal. Teamwork is a theme widely emphasized in our training and education throughout life.

In many years as an administrator, my biggest headache was employee relations. Why were those two always fighting about their sections? Why is there rivalry between the night shift and the morning shift, then the morning shift and the evening shift? The finger pointing between departments was widespread. The housekeepers blame the nurse aides, who blame the dietary staff, who blame the maintenance man, who blames the administrator, who blames the corporate office...why can't we all just get along and get the job done?

Do we spend more time accusing and talking about the problems than coming up with solutions and fixing what we can? Of course we need to get to the bottom of why we are running out of towels or finding puddles of water on the floor. Investigations must be conducted. Bad practices should be addressed. People must be accountable. Facts are facts. Gossip is gossip. Which do you spend more time on and what are your intentions?

> *...coworkers and supervisors at all levels would be wise to consider the importance of reciprocal interpersonal exchanges that enhance security, mutual respect, and positive feelings.* (Jennings 5)

Long-term care is dramatic. A substantial percentage of the people who live in assisted living and nursing homes feel they did not choose to be there. The families feel guilty for "putting them" in the care of others. Everyone is underpaid. The direct care staff, housekeepers and dietary staff do not make a livable wage. Many work two jobs and are barely keeping their heads above water financially. Fighting amongst ourselves compounds the problems we already have to wrestle. Integrity is about being accountable for what we produce and keeping our performance clean, regardless of how others conduct themselves.

Caregivers support personal growth when they teach each other better ways to work. When we share our strengths, despite the temptation to lay blame, we generate outcomes that are good for the whole care community. Show compassion for a co-worker who is struggling to learn the ropes, improve on time management or figure out what works. "To be dedicated to human spiritual development is to be dedicated to the race of which we are a part, and this therefore means dedication to our own development as well as 'theirs.'" (Peck 82)

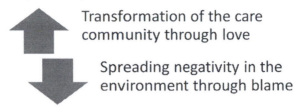

Transformation of the care community through love

Spreading negativity in the environment through blame

**Fig. 4.3** Which Arrow Do You Choose to Ride?

On behalf of those we serve and for our own sanity, we are going to heal this industry. To heal we get in touch with love. We forgive others of their trespasses and ask forgiveness for ours. To some, forgiveness is a sign of weakness or defeat.

*Throughout history, the way of love and truth has always won.*
Ghandi

Those who practice forgiveness know the freedom created when one truly forgives another. Those who forgive are liberated and made powerful—quite opposite from being stuck in conflict. No one loses anything by forgiving.

Our line of work is full of opportunities to disagree. People hold onto opinions, and there is widespread judgment about who is working harder than whom. The comparisons of better, faster, smarter, lazier, etc...need to go away. Let's hear "Nice going" and "We can do it." more often. Along with saying the words, start feeling the message. Finding fault with those around us is easy; far more useful is to concentrate on finding the positive. Once you are in the habit of seeking the good, saying the words and believing them will follow.

*Express approval of others,
appraise situations as good regardless
of appearances, and glorify your own
appearance and world. As you do,
you will become a part of the
resurrecting power of love.*
(Ponder 64)

When our minds are full of criticism, there is no room for love. When we only see the problems, we do not see the solutions. When we keep our thoughts loving and kind, we will experience our days as loving and kind, and our residents will feel our loving and kind energy.

Time and time again, problems that arise in every day caregiving are tests in love. Affirmations quoted in this section are tools for looking forward rather than hanging onto wrongs and errors. **Lack of cooperation amongst co-workers decreases productivity and is a disservice to our residents.**

Respect for differences, not absolute agreement, is the cornerstone of building solid work relationships. Improve on showing kindness and appreciation throughout the entire workplace. We will all be healthier when we practice loving our team members. What follows is a fabulous perspective for doing just that.

*I praise divine love that there
is a strong, wise way out of this
dilemma.*
(Ponder 24)

## I-Thou, I-You, I-It Relationships

While writing this book, I found a translation of the book *Ich und Du*, on my mother's book shelf. Written by Martin Buber in 1922, the book is referenced by Dr. Kitwood throughout *Dementia Reconsidered*. The German words, Ich and Du, translate to the words I and You or in some translations, I and Thou. Buber's philosophy of how we view and interact with others as I and You is a perfect fit for rementia theory.

The word thou is rarely used in modern speech, yet the concept of I–Thou communication is compellingly beautiful. Using thou evokes a sense of willing submission to a loving and powerful presence. In Walter Kaufman's translation of "I and Thou," the text replaces I–Thou with I–You. Both convey that in a loving human to human encounter, we regard the other as an equal. Unfortunately, often residents are forced into roles where they become non-equal, non-human. Buber refers to this as the "I–It" relationship. The similar concept was discussed earlier using Dr. Kitwood terms such as dehumanization and objectification.

Buber relays the difference between I–You and I–It as follows:

> Love is a cosmic force. For those who stand in it and behold in it, men emerge from their entanglement in busy-ness...Love is responsibility of an I for a You... (Buber 66)
>
> Every You in the world is doomed by nature to become a thing or at least to enter into thing-hood again and again. (Buber 69)

When caught in the busy 1-2-3, get it done work style, the caregiver to resident interaction becomes I–It, turning a human being into a non-feeling object. A person's need becomes a thing or action, a chore to be done. The more unbalanced the caregiver's workload, the more likely she will default to I–It relationships with residents.

Thinghood is the opposite of personhood. Love returns us to I–You, wherein the human being is rightly acknowledged. We demonstrate through loving words and actions that residents are worthy of our time, full attention, and dedication. The I–You relationship is one of the highest regard for another.

**The I–You relationship allows for graceful interaction.** Communicate with dignity for yourself and the one to whom you speak. Before saying it, ask yourself three questions:

> Is what I am about to say helpful?
> Is what I am about to say kind?
> Is what I am about to say true?

**The I–You relationship allows for grateful exchanges.** With gratitude for each position and every person, we acknowledge the glory of our relationships. Our co-workers and residents are treated with the utmost regard:

> I behold the goodness in you.
> I regard you as capable and qualified.
> My highest self recognizes your highest self.

As we see ourselves and others through the healing eyes of love, the I–You approach will become second nature. We are in the service of loving our residents above all else. "When we extend our limits through love, we do so by reaching out, so to speak, toward the beloved, whose growth we wish to nurture." (Peck 94)

Love creates success stories.

Faith, a 78 year old woman who had been living alone, was found "out of her mind" roaming through traffic completely nude. Two months after being in the nursing and rehabilitation facility, I took her to the local Miss Long-Term Care Beauty Pageant where she wowed the audience with her model looks in a long dress, high heels, and a boa. She sang "The Lady is a Tramp" for her talent performance. That's **rementia**—return to the highest self. Faye, who came to a nursing home disheveled and confused, was returned to her true essence with the care she could not give herself in her own home. The staff loved her outgoing personality. Her self-expression was encouraged, and she blossomed again into a lovely lady.

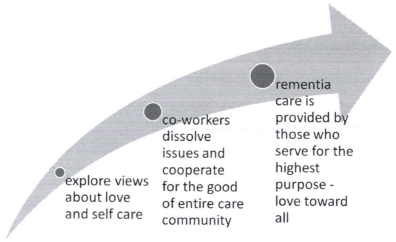

explore views about love and self care

co-workers dissolve issues and cooperate for the good of entire care community

rementia care is provided by those who serve for the highest purpose - love toward all

**Figure 4.4** Upward Bound

Caring for the aged is no longer only about keeping a body alive. Caring for a person with dementia is no longer just keeping a body safe. Caring is love, the center of human existence, the greatest of all gifts.

> Caregiving is not just about
> Now getting him out
> Of yesterday's well worn clothes
> Rementia is where
> Beyond the blank stare
> A future with a new plan grows

*When we love someone…we take an extra step or walk an extra mile. Love is not effortless. To the contrary, love is effortful. (Peck 83)*

# Bringing It All Together

Engagement, assistance, and love—the three components of rementia—are happening every day in care communities. *We can take it to the next level.* Rementia is an anticipated outcome.

Change does not come about easily. We can take bold yet careful steps. As awareness is raised with regard to how persons with dementia are perceived, we will move into an arena of caregiving that allows dignity for everyone involved. The more we expand limitations put on those with forms of dementia and ourselves as caregivers, the more equipped we are to become leaders in the ***person-centered care*** movement. We can cultivate the respect and recognition we have for so long deserved. As we give, so shall we receive.

The primary goal of *Getting REAL About Alzheimer's* is to spark dialogue about change so profound that caregivers will be praised as powerful people who achieve stellar results. *Getting REAL* can be taken in multiple directions with ideas from myriads of caregivers. When we are willing to go to great lengths, we can make history as the generation that transformed how long-term care is delivered.

# TILT Keys on Love

These questions are very personal and may evoke strong feelings. Some participants may not be comfortable sharing. That is okay.

1. Do you believe that your thoughts and words of love have power?

2. Which words below describe how you feel about the I–Thou, I–You approach?

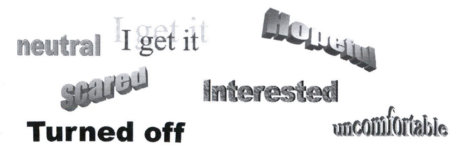

3. Does anything from your past prevent you from expressing love for your residents?

4. Recall a powerful experience involving appreciation amongst residents or co-workers.

5.  What would it take for you to release negative beliefs about your workplace?

6.  Think of a specific example of how can you foster team work.

7.  Do you have symptoms of job burnout? Can you describe this?

8.  Are you open to the transformation process?

9.  What do you think of the term "healer?"

10. What is the greatest lesson you have learned from this guide?

# References

## Dictionaries

*The American Heritage*, Fourth Edition. New York: Dell Publishing a division of Random House, Inc. 2001. Print.

*The Merriam Webster Dictionary*, New Edition. Massachusetts: Merriam-Webster, Incorporated. 2004. Print.

*Webster's New Dictionary of the English Language*. New York: The Popular Group, LLC. 2005. Print.

## Books

Buber, Martin. I and Thou, A New Translation with prologue and notes by Walter Kaufman. New York: Charles Scribner's Sons, 1970. Print.

Feel, Naomi. The Validation Breakthrough. Maryland: Health Professions Press, Inc., 1993. Print.

Kitwood, Tom. Dementia Reconsidered: The Person Comes First. New York: Open University Press, 1997. Print.

Ondaatje, Michael. The English Patient. New York: Vintage Books, a Division of Random House, Inc., 1992. Print.

Peale, Norman. Why Some Positive Thinkers Get Powerful Results. New York: Foundation for Christian Living, 1986. Print.

Peck, M. Scott. The Road Less Travelled. New York: Simon & Schuster, 1978. Print.

Ponder, Catherine. The Prospering Power of Love. California: DeVorss & Company, 1966. Print.

Simard, Joyce. The End of Life Namaste Care Program. Maryland: Health Professions Press, Inc., 2007. Print.

# Articles

Buettner, Linda. Legg, Timothy. "Activities: What is Appropriate?" in *Provider*, Mar 2012: p 43-48.

Lourde, Kathleen. "Bridging the Gap in Dementia Care" in *Provider*, Sept 2012: p 22-32.

Lourde, Kathleen. "Open Minds, Open Hearts: English Rose Suites' Dementia Care Philosophy" in *Provider*, Sept 2012: p 28-30

Tucker, Jennifer. "A Dementia Care Revolution" in *Provider*, Nov 2012: p 43-45.

# Websites

Jennings, BM. Work Stress and Burnout Among Nurses: Role of the Work Environment and Working Conditions. In: Hughes RG, editor. Patient Safety and Quality: An Evidence-Based Handbook for Nurses. Rockville (MD): Agency for Healthcare Research and Quality (US); Apr 2008, Chapter 26. Available from: http://www.ncbi.nlm.nih.gov/books/NBK2668/. Date of access Nov 2013. Web.

Serafin, Jennifer. "Bathing How-To's for the Elderly." www.caring.com. Date of access Dec 2013, Web.

Taylor, Edgar. Edwards, Marian. "The Old Man and His Grandson." Fairy Tales by the Grimm Brothers. Authorama. www.authorama.com. Date of access: Oct 2013. Web.

Website with no specific quote or citation: www. alz.org

Author's website: Alzheimer's Connection La Mesa,
www.alzconnectlamesa.com

# About the Author

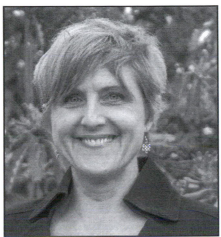

Photo by Russel Ray Photography

Kassandra A. King, BA, NHA, RCFE

Kassandra King's involvement with the geriatric population began in her early teen years as a volunteer with The Holiday Project and with her high school choir. She has always enjoyed the company and wisdom of her elders in long-term care settings and has a natural ability to relate to those with Alzheimer's disease and other forms of dementia. She holds a bachelor's degree from the University of North Texas and post graduate certification in long-term care from Texas State University. She began her professional tour of duty as a licensed administrator in 1996, gaining vast experience at several large facilities in Texas and California.

Holding the torch for education and awareness, Ms. King has served at two chapters of the Alzheimer's Association in the capacity of Public Policy Director and Professional Education Manager. Her inspiration to write this book came about from her work as a Program Manager of Engagement at one of the largest memory care communities in California. She is the owner of Alzheimer's Connection La Mesa, where she is happily occupied as a care consultant, care manager, and dementia care educator.

Ms. King is the mother of two extraordinary young men who have spent many hours waiting for her to finish making rounds, and who read to residents, entertained them by playing guitar, and joined in Christmas Eve caroling. She is currently the San Diego East County Locality coordinator for The Holiday Project.